HOW TO S
STANDARDIZED TESTS

DONALD J. SEFCIK, DO, MBA

Director of Academic Innovation and Psychometrics
Senior Associate Dean
Professor
Michigan State University
College of Osteopathic Medicine
East Lansing, Michigan

GILLIAN BICE, PhD

Director of Academic and Professional Development
Assistant Professor
Adjunct Professor of Anthropology
Michigan State University
College of Osteopathic Medicine
East Lansing, Michigan

FRANK PREROST, PhD

Professor
Department of Family Medicine
Midwestern University
College of Osteopathic Medicine
Downers Grove, Illinois

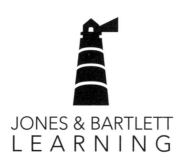

JONES & BARTLETT
LEARNING

World Headquarters
Jones & Bartlett Learning
5 Wall Street
Burlington, MA 01803
978-443-5000
info@jblearning.com
www.jblearning.com

Jones & Bartlett Learning books and products are available through most bookstores and online booksellers. To contact Jones & Bartlett Learning directly, call 800-832-0034, fax 978-443-8000, or visit our website, www.jblearning.com.

Substantial discounts on bulk quantities of Jones & Bartlett Learning publications are available to corporations, professional associations, and other qualified organizations. For details and specific discount information, contact the special sales department at Jones & Bartlett Learning via the above contact information or send an email to specialsales@jblearning.com.

Some images in this book feature models. These models do not necessarily endorse, represent, or participate in the activities represented in the images.

This publication is designed to provide accurate and authoritative information in regard to the Subject Matter covered. It is sold with the understanding that the publisher is not engaged in rendering legal, accounting, or other professional service. If legal advice or other expert assistance is required, the service of a competent professional person should be sought.

Production Credits
Publisher: William Brottmiller
Acquisitions Editor: Katey Birtcher
Managing Editor: Maro Gartside
Editorial Assistant: Teresa Reilly
Editorial Assistant: Kayla Dos Santos
Production Assistant: Rebekah Linga
Marketing Manager: Grace Richards
Manufacturing and Inventory Control
  Supervisor: Amy Bacus
Composition: Laserwords Private Limited, Chennai, India
Cover Design: Scott Moden
Cover Image: Students studying with laptops: © Diego Cervo/ShutterStock, Inc.; Scantron test sheet: © Artifan/ShutterStock, Inc.
Printing and Binding: Malloy, Inc.
Cover Printing: Malloy, Inc.

Library of Congress Cataloging-in-Publication Data
Sefcik, Donald J.
  How to study for standardized tests / Donald J. Sefcik, Frank Prerost, and Gillian Bice.
    p. cm.
  Includes bibliographical references and index.
  ISBN 978-0-7637-7362-5 (pbk.) — ISBN 0-7637-7362-X (ibid.)
  1. Test-taking skills. 2. Examinations—Study guides. 3. Achievement tests—Study guides. 4. Educational tests and measurements—Study guides. I. Prerost, Frank. II. Bice, Gillian. III. Title.
  LB3060.57.S45 2013
  371.26—dc23
                                                                                    2011044596

6048

Printed in the United States of America
16 15 14 13   10 9 8 7 6 5 4 3 2

Table of Contents

Part

1

Preparing for Your Test

Section

I

Chapter

1

Reviewers

Craig S. Boisvert, DO
Professor
West Virginia School of Osteopathic
  Medicine
Lewisburg, WV

Cynthia Bunde, MPAS, PA-C
Physician Assistant Studies
Idaho State University
Pocatello, ID

Cristy Daniel, MS, OTR/L
Assistant Professor and Academic
  Fieldwork Coordinator
College of Saint Mary
Omaha, NE

**Emily J. Davidson, BS, RPA-C,
  DC**
Associate Professor, Associate
  Director
Physician Assistant Program
City University New York—York
  College
Jamaica, NY

Laura R. Durbin, RN, BSN, CHPN
Instructor
West Kentucky Community and
  Technical College
Paducah, KY

Carol W. Ennulat, MBA, PA-C
Assistant Director, Assistant
  Professor, Academic
  Coordinator
Physician Assistant Studies Program
Chatham University
Pittsburgh, PA

Gail Feinberg, DO, FACOFP
Regional Assistant Dean
West Virginia School of
  Osteopathic Medicine
Lewisburg, WV

Kristin B. Haas, OTR/L, MOT, OTD
Assistant Professor
College of Saint Mary
Omaha, NE

Bernadette Howlett, PhD
Research Assistant Professor
Physician Assistant Studies
Idaho State University
Pocatello, ID

**Norma Krumwiede, EdD, MEd,
  MN, RN**
Professor
Minnesota State University,
  Mankato
Mankato, MN

John E. Lopes, Jr., DHSc, PA-C
Assistant Professor
Physician Assistant Program
Central Michigan University
Mount Pleasant, MI

John O'Hare, MS, RT (R)
Long Island University
Brookville, NY

Catherine B. Pearman, MPAS, PA-C
Physician Assistant Program
Eastern Virginia Medical School
Norfolk, VA

Joan Pollner, MSN, RN, CHPN
Director of Nurse Education
Warren County Community College
Washington, NJ

Denise Rizzolo, PA-C, PhD
Assistant Clinical Professor
Physician Assistant Program
Pace University-Lenox Hill Hospital
New York, NY

Thomas J. Yarcheski, PhD
Professor and Program Coordinator
Health Services Administration
Keiser University
Fort Lauderdale, FL

About the Authors

Donald Sefcik, DO, MBA, is director of academic innovation and psychometrics and senior associate dean at the Michigan State University College of Osteopathic Medicine (MSUCOM), East Lansing. Dr. Sefcik holds a BS degree in pharmacy and an MS degree in pharmacology from Butler University, Indianapolis, Indiana, and an MBA from Purdue University, Hammond, Indiana. Don started teaching in 1981 and has been involved in the education of osteopathic (DO) medical students; allopathic (MD) medical students; pharmacy, nursing, and physician assistant students; as well as a wide variety of undergraduate students considering various professional degrees. Dr. Sefcik has particular interests in study techniques, student-centered teaching, and remediation practices. He is board certified in both family practice and emergency medicine. Active in a large number of professional organizations and committees, Dr. Sefcik has received numerous awards for his teaching.

Gillian Bice, PhD, is the director of academic and professional development at the Michigan State University College of Osteopathic Medicine. Dr. Bice holds a BS in zoology, as well as an MA and PhD in physical anthropology, all from Michigan State University. Before joining the faculty of MSUCOM, Dr. Bice was manager and supervisor of the MSU Clinical Cytogenetics Laboratory. Since 1995, Dr. Bice has been teaching anthropology and anatomy courses to undergraduate, graduate, and graduate-professional students. In her current role, Dr. Bice advises medical students on issues pertaining to best learning practices and career development.

Frank Prerost, PhD, is a professor in the Department of Family Medicine at Midwestern University Chicago College of Osteopathic Medicine. Dr. Prerost holds PhD and MA degrees in clinical psychology from DePaul University, Chicago, Illinois, and a BS degree in behavioral science from the University of Illinois. Previously, Dr. Prerost was program director of the Behavioral Medicine Department at Midwestern University, Downers Grove, Illinois, and director of the Midwestern Geriatric Education Center. For many years, Dr. Prerost has been extensively involved in the education and training of students in osteopathic medicine, clinical psychology, gerontology, and physician assistant studies. He is a licensed clinical psychologist and certified through the National Register of Health Service Providers in psychology. Dr. Prerost is a seasoned researcher who has published in many professional journals and has also authored a number of instructor manuals to facilitate student learning.

Roadmap of This Book

Standardized test scores are the result of the interaction between preparation and performance. This can be expressed as the following formula:

$$Score = f(preparation + performance)$$

Furthermore

Test preparation includes all the variables and activities that define test-wiseness (TW). Test performance includes all the variables and activities that define test-taking skills (TTS).

Therefore

$$Score = f(TW + TTS)$$

Part 1 of this book presents, describes, and explains TW, which focuses on three key variables: the test, you and various study resources, and methods and techniques.

Figure FM-1

Roadmap

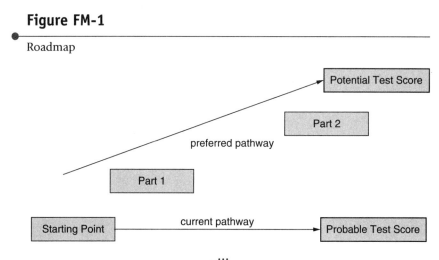

Part 2 of this book presents, describes, and explains TTS, which includes how to work most effectively and efficiently in a timed environment, techniques that will help you select the best answers, and ways to reduce the impact of test anxiety.

Each section and its associated chapters build on and contribute to the previous material. This book begins by presenting the basics elements of test-wiseness (Part 1) and concludes with test-taking skills (Part 2). This roadmap will help you navigate the pathway to a higher test score. We recommend reading this book from beginning to end.

Introduction

High examination scores result from two factors: optimal preparation *before* the test and optimal performance *during* the test. Perhaps that's too obvious, but it's really that simple. However, the other part of the equation is that there's frequently a wide chasm that separates what we know from what we actually do. The purpose of this book is to help you build a bridge to cross that chasm and transform your knowledge into action.

At its most basic level, this book is about two concepts: test-wiseness and test-taking skills (Lai & Waltman, 2008; Mahamed, Gregory, & Austin, 2006; Milman, Bishop, & Ebel, 1965; Morse, 1998; Samson, 1985; Scruggs & Mastropieri, 1992; Slakter, Koehler, & Hampton, 1970). Test-wiseness means knowing as much as you possibly can about your upcoming test and using this information effectively and efficiently to become well prepared *prior* to test day. Having successfully done that, achieving mastery of an array of test-taking skills will allow you to perform on test day at the level of test-taking expert.

If you prepare *and* perform to the level of your capability, it is our contention that you will do quite well. Reading this book isn't sufficient—it's not a magic book—but by learning as much as you can about what it takes to perform well on standardized tests and by following our recommendations you can realize your high-scoring potential. This truly is the road less traveled. The vast majority of standardized test-takers do not avail themselves of this level of personal development, but we hope you will accept the challenge and join us on the journey.

Why should you buy a book on how to study for multiple-choice question tests?

1. You want to increase your test score.
2. You believe that although you will perform well, you can do better.
3. You want to learn how to study less and still get a high score.
4. You are committed to devoting the time and energy necessary to improve your study techniques and test-taking skills.
5. All of the above.

If you selected none of the above, then please place this book back on the shelf; purchasing this book will provide no value for you (unless you're buying it as a gift). If you selected option 5 (all of the above), then proceed to checkout. If you chose any of options 1–4, read a bit further; this might be the book for you.

How do you *feel* about taking a comprehensive, standardized test?

The thought of taking a comprehensive, standardized test is terrifying for many and can induce paralytic fear in some. The reality is that to achieve your career goals, not only will you be taking the examination, but you will likely need to do well on one or more major "gateway" exams. Whether you need to take the Graduate Record Examination, the Medical College Admissions Test, the Law School Admissions Test, or any other aptitude test, as well as comprehensive course examinations or certificate or licensure examinations, the reality is that a standardized test or two (or more) looms in your future.

Perhaps the thought doesn't put you into a state of panic—sweaty palms, racing heart, visit to the emergency room (one of us has been there, done that; another of us has been there, seen it . . . many times)—but simply a state of heightened arousal. Maybe you don't know where to start or how to begin, or you've had a prior bad experience with a standardized exam (like the ACT or the SAT). Maybe you just know you can do better and need a little boost to get you where you want to be. Whatever the reason, we're confident we can help.

Why do people fear comprehensive, standardized exams?

Why do people fail these exams or fail to perform as well as they could?

The first question is easy to answer. People fear these exams because there's generally a lot riding on them. A lot of this is psychological. Excessive anxiety about exam performance can stem from low self-esteem, low self-efficacy, fear of failure, fear of rejection by loved ones, fear of success, fear of the unknown, anxiety disorders, and a host of other reasons. However, there's also the very real fact of consequences. Failing a big exam can throw a wrench into your life plans, making it difficult or nearly impossible to progress in or toward your career, and costing you time and money in your effort to retake the exam. Thus, there are legitimate reasons to be anxious, but the point is to not allow the situation to get out of control. Furthermore, it's not necessarily the anxiety itself that is the source of the problem, but rather how you deal with it. Some anxiety is healthy and motivational, but too much is crippling.

It's important to have a realistic outlook regarding the importance of the exam and the consequence of failure, as well as a good set of coping mechanisms to deal with excessive anxiety. This book will spend a fair bit of time addressing the issue of test anxiety and how it can impact studying for and taking exams. We will help you understand the important role of emotions in test performance and offer guidance and several solutions to many of the most common obstacles to success, such as test anxiety and procrastination.

The answer to the second question—why do people fail exams or fail to perform well—is complicated, but generally there are two reasons:

1. Failure to adequately prepare
2. Failure to adequately execute

Many kinds of problems fall under the heading of "failure to adequately prepare," including:

- Fundamental lack of content knowledge
- Bad time management
- Inadequate time to prepare
- Poor planning
- Inadequate study/learning strategies and techniques
- Inadequate type or amount of practice
- Misunderstanding the exam format or content

Even if one has adequately prepared, failure to adequately execute on exam day can produce an unacceptably low score. Poor execution can also stem from a variety of sources including:

- Inadequate reading skills
- Poor reasoning skills
- Cognitive errors and biases
- Poor time management during the exam
- Test anxiety
- Lack of test-taking skills

It is not uncommon for people who are about to sit for a potentially life-altering exam to enter the process completely unaware of the tremendous number of variables that might affect their score, or who believe that all it takes to do well on an exam is to buy the most popular review book and try to memorize its contents. You may even believe this is true because you've talked to someone who told you that's what they did. Maybe what they told you is partly or even mostly true—for them—but what you don't know is how all the other variables came into play. Maybe this person thinks they simply memorized the review book, but they actually had more content knowledge to begin with, or maybe they have exceptional reading skills or reasoning skills. Maybe they're a "good test-taker." Perhaps they didn't tell you everything else they did to prepare, or maybe they're just plain smarter than you are. The point is everyone is different, and you need to do what is right for you, not what worked for someone else. That is precisely where this book excels and others fall flat. It's not about telling you what's the best thing for you to do; it's about helping you discover that for yourself by teaching you how to acquire the tools, skills, and strategies you will need in order to learn more and then show what you know (and maybe show more than you know) on an exam.

How does this book differ from existing test preparation resources and review courses?

Collectively, the authors have over 70 years of experience working with examinees—undergraduate, graduate, and graduate-professional students studying for a wide array of examinations—helping them achieve higher scores. Some of those we've worked with—even those with multiple failures on a national standardized exam—have increased their performance by over two standard deviations. That's equivalent to moving from a failing score to one above the 70th percentile.

Far too many review books and courses focus on content alone. Many others rely on gimmicks; their focus is more on marketing a product that purports to increase your test score and make studying easier rather than helping you understand how to learn and develop the transferable skills you need to achieve a higher score, not just on one specific exam but all exams. We're not going to sugarcoat it. It takes work. It takes time. It takes planning. It's not easy and there are no shortcuts (but there are evidence-based methods and strategies demonstrated to improve efficiency and effectiveness!).

What factors account for people who routinely tend to score high versus low on exams?

Some of the factors that account for differences between high and low scorers include:

- Dynamic/strategic planning versus "winging it"
- Frequent self-assessment with appropriate strategic adjustments
- Use of active versus passive learning techniques

- Studying to problem solve versus memorizing (i.e., use of deep versus superficial learning techniques)
- Use of effective and efficient study techniques and avoidance of time wasters
- Preparing for the type of exam to be taken (i.e., a comprehensive, standardized multiple-choice exam)

Preparing for a high-stakes, comprehensive examination requires you to actively and simultaneously manage several variables:

- *Time*: You will need to prioritize and schedule (e.g., when you will study, for how long, and how your studying will interface with your other obligations, needs, and desires).
- *Effort*: You will need to allocate the appropriate level of effort into areas that will maximize your test score.
- *Attitude*: You will need to develop a positive outlook in approaching the exam.
- *Motivation*: You will need to develop effective techniques to keep your motivation level as high as possible throughout the process. Most everyone experiences periods of time in which studying seems nearly impossible because their emotional reserves are on "empty." Emotional and physical well-being cannot be overrated—they are simply vital to maintaining higher cognitive functioning.
- *Selections*: You will need to choose your study aids (determine what you will study) and your study behaviors (determine how you will study).

Notice that when you combine the first letters of each of the variables it spells out the word TEAMS.

Before delving further, let's revisit our first question: Why buy a book on how to study for multiple-choice question tests? If you chose option 1 (because you want to increase your test score), then you recognize you can be more effective. That's great, you have a goal. If you chose option 2 (because you believe that although you will perform well, you can do better), then you possess a quality known as self-efficacy. Good—examinees that possess this trait can learn to study better and score higher on examinations! If you chose option 3 (you want to learn how you can study less and still get a high score), then you are interested in learning to be more efficient. We can help with that! If you chose option 4 (you are committed to devoting the time and energy necessary to improve your study techniques and test-taking skills), then you are motivated and ready to become a more self-regulated learner. If you chose option 6 (all of the above), then this is the book for you.

By following the advice is this book, you will be better prepared for your examination. This book is our invitation to you to change or enhance your current study techniques. This book will help you understand what you can, should, and must do, which, in a nutshell, is to become a more effective learner. This book was written for one purpose—to increase the test scores of everyone that takes a multiple-choice test.

To accomplish this goal, the book is divided into two parts and four sections:

Part 1: Preparing for Your Test (Developing Test-Wiseness)
    Section I: Understanding Your Opponent (The Test)
    Section II: Developing Your T.E.A.M.S.
    Section III: Practicing Your Skills
Part 2: Taking Your Test (Applying Test-Taking Skills)
    Section IV: Executing Your Game Plan (Test Day)

Where should you focus your studying?

How much time should you allocate to studying?

How should you begin studying?

What are the best study techniques to use to increase your test scores?

How can you improve your ability to remember facts?

How do you know if your plan is working?

The answers to these questions and many more can be found in the chapters that follow.

To help guide and promote improvement in your study techniques and test scores, we included a series of *Exercises* and *Activities* throughout this book. Prior to reading Chapter 1, please complete Exercises 1 and 2.

EXERCISES AND ACTIVITIES

Becoming competent in the performance of any skill is based on two key elements: knowledge and practice. First, you have to know what it is you need to do (i.e., you need *knowledge*). Once you know what is required, then you need to *practice* doing it until you do it well. Once you are competent, the challenge shifts from being able to do it to doing it at the appropriate times. Sounds so simple, right? Then why is it so difficult to do?

Speizer (2005) reported that 80–90% of traditional training programs result in little to no change in overall performance. Rackham (1979) reported that almost 90% of new skills gained in training programs are lost just four weeks after the training program ends. We want you to do much better. We want you to improve your performance and continue to do so after you have gained the new skill. To help you accomplish this we created a series of exercises and activities that are presented throughout this book.

We define exercises and activities as follows:

- *Exercises* are mental challenges. Exercises will be found prior to a section or chapter. They are designed to engage your mind and cause you to think about a concept.
  - o   What do you know or believe?
  - o   What do you value?
  - o   How would you approach a situation?
- *Activities* are practice opportunities. Activities will be found after a chapter or section. They are designed to reinforce a principle or concept through reflection and some action or actions.
  - o   Did you appreciate the key concepts in the chapter?
  - o   Where will you apply the discussed concepts to practice them?
  - o   How will you internalize what you learned?
  - o   What will your next steps be?

The exercises and activities that you will encounter throughout the book offer you an opportunity to start to change your thinking, behaviors, and skills. Choosing not to complete them is a choice that you might make. We hope that you choose to complete them all, in order. We are confident that doing so will serve you well.

EXERCISE 1

Drafting Your Study Plan (V1)

We want you to get the highest score on your test that you can. To assist you in the development of a study plan, the first thing you need to do is identify what your current mind-set is about the task before you (i.e., the standardized test that you will be taking). What are your current thoughts about the test? How do you plan to study? What resources will you use? This exercise is designed to make your current plan concrete—you need to write it down so that you can examine it, expand it, and improve it as you read the remaining chapters of this book. Please see Table FM-1, which contains Exercise 1.

Many examinees have strong emotional feelings about upcoming tests. We want to help you examine your feelings. We want your plan to be realistic and based on evidence, not well-intentioned opinions or intuition. You need to write your thoughts down so that as you read this book you can review, modify, and enhance your plan.

Table	
FM-1	Exercise 1

Questions

1. Why am I planning to take this test?

2. What study techniques will I use to prepare for this test?

3. Which books, computer programs, study aids, etc., will I use to help me prepare?

4. How much total time will I study for this test; how long will I study each day?

5. When will I start studying for this test?

6. What can I do on the day of the test to increase my score?

7. As the test approaches, how will I know that I am getting ready?

Answer the seven questions that follow. In the ensuing chapters, we present what the literature reports and share what our experiences have taught us about test preparation and test-taking. We offer suggestions and recommendations for you to consider as you learn more about standardized tests and how to prepare for them. Your seven answers create your first draft of a study plan (V1 = Version 1). It is our hope that your answers will change a few times before you complete this book. When you complete the book your final exercise will be the creation of your final study plan.

EXERCISE 2

What Kind of Exam-Preparer Am I?

Test scores can be divided into three simple categories: very low, average, and very high. Although not absolute, educational psychology and cognitive research have identified behaviors and skills sets that are more commonly observed in high achievers—those that get the highest test scores. How many of these characteristics do you possess? In which of these behaviors do you most commonly engage?

Table FM-2 enumerates some common study behaviors and skills sets. Each statement should be rated on the following scale: Almost never; Sometimes; Almost always. For each, select your typical behavior—*do not answer* based on what you are familiar with or what you generally intend to do. Answer each item based on what you actually do. *Be brutally honest.* Only you will review your answers.

Table FM-3 depicts the "best" selections for each item based on the literature and our experience. The rationale for each response is discussed in the chapters that follow.

Table		Almost Always	Sometimes	Almost Never
FM–2	Exercise 2, Part 1			
Behavior				
1.	I study until the last possible minute before my test starts.			
2.	I highlight important material in my book so that I can find it later.			
3.	I often text or answer emails during my study sessions.			
4.	I study several hours only right before the test.			
5.	My goal is to study as little as possible without lowering my grade.			
6.	I often draw my own pictures and create tables when I study.			
7.	When I study I focus on things that I need to do to avoid failing.			
8.	I study material until I can reproduce it from memory.			
9.	I start studying long before the test.			
10.	I study with music on in the background.			
11.	I use flash cards as my primary study aid.			
12.	When I study, I write questions that I could be asked on the test.			
13.	I use a few good study techniques for most of my studying needs.			
14.	I often add notes to the margins of my books and class notes.			
15.	A review book or summary guide is my primary study resource.			

Table FM–3	Exercise 2, Part 2	Almost Always	Sometimes	Almost Never
Behavior				
1.	I study until the last possible minute before my test starts.			X
2.	I highlight important material in my book so that I can find it later.		X	
3.	I often text or answer emails during my study sessions.			X
4.	I study several hours only right before the test.			X
5.	My goal is to study as little as possible without lowering my grade.			X
6.	I often draw my own pictures and create tables when I study.	X		
7.	When I study I focus on things that I need to do to avoid failing.			X
8.	I study material until I can reproduce it from memory.		X	
9.	I start studying long before the test.	X		
10.	I study with music on in the background.			X
11.	I use flash cards as my primary study aid.			X
12.	When I study, I write questions that I could be asked on the test.	X		
13.	I use a few good study techniques for most of my studying needs.	X		
14.	I often add notes to the margins of my books and class notes.	X		
15.	A review book or summary guide is my primary study resource.		X	

Acknowledgments

As with all projects that require several years to complete, the final product is the result of significant input and support from many individuals.

To MaryLee Davis, PhD; Lindsay Boik-Price, DO; and Danielle Harik (MSUCOM Class of 2014). We wish to offer special thanks for proofreading multiple versions of this text, as well as for your great ideas and candid, insightful feedback. We will be eternally grateful for these exceptional individuals. Without their efforts this book would not have reached its final form.

To our patient and tireless supporters: Elizabeth, Jo Ann, John, Mimi, and Scott. Thanks for always being there and for understanding that sometimes our passion reduces our availability.

To our many subliminal contributors. Although we referenced many works in our book, we are confident that many authors—whom we inadvertently have not cited—have significantly, and perhaps unconsciously, influenced us over the years. We wish to thank you all collectively. Any citation omissions are truly unintentional.

To all of you who have helped us gain an appreciation for what we do and taught us how to do it better—our teachers, students, coaches, mentors, and critics. We are most appreciative and wish to sincerely thank you.

Part

1

Preparing for Your Test (Developing Test-Wiseness)

I Understanding Your Opponent (The Test)

YOU NEED A GAME PLAN!

A guide to exam preparation wouldn't be worth much if it didn't provide you with insight into foundational concepts related to tests and study plans. In fact, this is the primary focus of section I. First, as a warm-up, we offer a time-honored analogy as a means of framing our discussion on test preparation: Studying for a test is like preparing for a competitive sporting event. You *need* a game plan.

A competition presents an opponent with multiple challenges to confront: time, distance, strength, endurance, skill level, effort, focus, and practice. As a contender, what would be your approach to determining the outcome of a competition?

1. Would you *hope* that good fortune smiles down on you to ensure your win?
2. Would you *believe* you are the superior contender who will prevail over your opponent with minimal preparation?
3. Would you *rationalize* your loss after the fact?
4. Or, would you *take control* and create a game plan—identify your weaknesses, schedule training (practice) sessions to hone your skills, and increase your strength and endurance—to maximize the probability of your victory?

HOW *DO* ELITE ATHLETES PREPARE FOR A SPORTING EVENT?

In our opinion, when elite athletes prepare they:

- study their opponent—understand what they are up against.
- understand the game—they know the rules.
- assess their own status as a competitor—they know their strengths and weaknesses.
- prepare physically—work out, practice, and develop important skills.
- prepare mentally—gain confidence in abilities and develop a winning attitude.
- develop a "game plan" for game day.

Getting ready for a test is quite similar. The main difference is the emphasis on mental activities and skills as opposed to physical. As a test-taker, your plan should involve the following:

1. familiarizing yourself with the test (get to know your "opponent")—review the rules, know what will be covered, anticipate the sorts of questions you will be asked,
2. assessing and reassessing your abilities (evaluate your skills, talents and level of knowledge), and of course,
3. improving your knowledge and skills by studying the appropriate content, completing practice questions, and developing test-wiseness and test-taking skills.

A fringe benefit of utilizing a methodical and organized approach to exam preparation—one that includes all the facets discussed above—is that you will likely increase your self-efficacy. You will come to believe that you do indeed have control over the variables that affect your test performance (i.e., your score). Test preparation is a multifaceted, iterative process that includes management of several variables (remember in the introduction, we introduced the acronym TEAMS: time, effort, attitude, motivation, selection).

Are you ready to start planning for a big win (high score) on exam day? We're sure you are, so keep reading.

1 Standardized Tests

THERE IS NO SUCH THING AS A "POOR STANDARDIZED TEST-TAKER"

In our opinion, anyone who has ever uttered the sentence, "I'm not a good standardized test-taker" should have said, "I don't prepare well for standardized tests." Our hope is that after reading this book you will have no need to say either.

We do not believe there is any such thing as a "poor standardized test-taker." The phrase itself creates the impression of a mysterious innate quality (or lack thereof) that renders someone constitutionally incapable of taking a standardized test. In our experience, students often offer this as an explanation for a low score, and they do so in a manner that is almost matter-of-fact and fatalistic as though that's just it, game over, they're bad at taking standardized tests, and they always will be because it's . . . part . . . of . . . who . . . they . . . *are*!

Certainly, standardized tests pose different challenges than other types of tests you have taken. However, there is no fundamental skill required for taking and doing well on a standardized test that you cannot master. It's all about proper preparation, and that's something you can do, with some guidance.

It's likely you've already taken a standardized test, such as the SAT or ACT, and you've probably talked with others about standardized tests. So, the first of many questions we will pose is this: What makes a standardized test a standardized test?

Do you know? Do you have an idea or a guess?

Don't read any further until you stop and think about your answer!

Do you have an answer yet? If yes, continue reading to see how your answer compares to ours. If not, reflect for a few moments more before proceeding.

Critical Comment: Active reflection is a valuable skill to develop. You should train yourself to periodically stop reading and think about the material. Ask and answer your own questions. How is this material related to what I already know? What is its relevance? This is a learning method called elaboration, and it is associated with deeper learning and better long-term memory retention (for more information, refer to Chapter 7).

Our answer: A standardized test differs from other types in its purpose and design. The ultimate purpose of a standardized test is, as the name implies, standardization; it provides a standard for comparison. Standardized tests are designed to evaluate and then compare the aptitudes or competencies of a diverse population of individuals (e.g., students from different institutions who have different educational backgrounds). Therefore, a standardized test must be: (1) representative of a domain of knowledge, (2) dependable with regard to the format and scoring, and (3) consistent in terms of testing conditions (*Standardized Assessment: A Primer*, 2011).

Critical Comment: If ever a word is unfamiliar to you, no matter what you're reading, be sure to look up the definition in a dictionary. Vocabulary is often tested on standardized exams. Don't memorize words and hope that you will recognize them on the test. Understand what you are studying—give it meaning! Incorporate new vocabulary into your everyday conversations. Make it fun. Stump your friends. Subscribe to a word-a-day service.

So, the question is: What is it about these qualities of standardized tests that makes them more challenging than the majority of exams and quizzes you have experienced thus far? To appreciate the answer to that question, you need a basic understanding of several aspects of test design.

TEACHER-GENERATED TESTS VERSUS STANDARDIZED TESTS

Teacher-generated tests are generally designed to evaluate your learning of the course material in order to assign a course grade. They are usually written for a specific course (e.g., BS101) within a specific discipline (e.g., bioscience) and are typically administered in the same classroom as the course is taught under the supervision of the faculty member responsible for teaching that course. The focus of teacher-generated exams is limited in content and the questions tend to emphasize knowledge of facts, specific details or specific concepts. They are generally not intended to measure learning across different courses or disciplines. In other words, if you take an exam in course SOS202 (social science), you are not likely to be tested on content you learned in a previous bioscience course (BS101) or history, chemistry, or algebra course unless that content was specifically covered in SOS202.

For teacher-generated course exams, the similarities or continuities between the learning environment and the testing environment provide numerous conscious and subconscious clues and memory cues (triggers) to help you recall information on the exam. For example, you might remember the sound of the professor's voice as she was explaining the concept you need to understand to answer a test question. Or you might visualize the professor standing in the front of the room explaining his PowerPoint slide to the class, which then triggers your recall of the correct answer to the question.

In contrast, standardized tests are designed to measure knowledge across courses, subjects, and disciplines; therefore, they generally cover a much broader domain of information. Their focus tends to be more global with an emphasis on associations, integration, and application (see Figure 1-1). They may even be intended to evaluate specific cognitive skills, such as problem solving, verbal reasoning, or analytical thinking. Moreover, standardized test questions are written and edited by a group of content experts and professional editors—people you have never met—using established test construction techniques developed with the intent of reducing your ability to use cues and clues to select the correct answers.

Finally, the questions themselves usually differ between the two types of exams. Test questions can be categorized by the type of cognitive task

Figure 1-1

The Two Primary Types of Tests

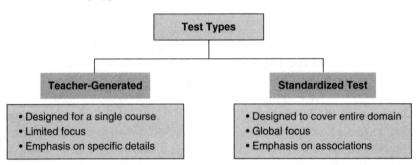

required to answer them. In the simplest sense, they are divided into two groups: low-level items or high-level items. Coursework frequently focuses on new terms, facts, and concepts. To assess a student's ability to recognize a term or recall a fact, teacher-generated tests generally ask questions that are limited in scope, depth, and complexity. Such questions are referred to as low-level thinking items. High-level thinking items require a deeper understanding of principles and concepts; they test the examinee's ability to solve a problem, evaluate a situation, make a judgment, or synthesize new ideas. In contrast to teacher-generated tests, standardized tests tend to be composed of a much higher percentage of high-level questions (see Figure 1-2). This tends to make standardized tests more challenging, especially if you're not expecting this difference.

Figure 1-2

The Two Basic Types of Test Questions

Test Questions

Lower-Level Thinking
- Designed to assess memory
- Focus on recognition
- Emphasis on specific details

Higher-Level Thinking
- Designed to assess problem-solving
- Focus on application in new situations
- Emphasis on critical reasoning

Many students learn to prepare for and perform on teacher-generated exams using just a few basic skills:

- Read and memorize key words or phrases from the textbook.
- Memorize class handouts and notes.
- Listen for clues from the teacher about what will likely be on the test.
- Memorize old test questions.
- Answer multiple-choice questions by recognizing memorized facts and concepts.
- Answer multiple-choice questions by recognizing clues provided by the teacher.

The bottom line is that through years of conditioning you have learned how to pass teacher-dependent, teacher-created tests. Standardized tests are teacher-*independent* tests. Excelling on standardized tests requires that you develop new skills and refine old skills. In short, you need to become a test-wise person with excellent test-taking skills. Before we follow that train of thought, we want to be sure you are familiar with a few more terms and concepts related to tests—validity, reliability, and scoring.

TEST VALIDITY AND RELIABILITY

A "good" test should possess two characteristics—validity and reliability. To be valid, the test must measure what it intends to measure. To be reliable, a test must produce essentially the same results when administered at multiple sites over an extended period of time; in other words, the results must be reproducible. A test that produces statistically different scores depending on the testing location is not reliable. A test cannot be valid if it is not also reliable.

There are several types of validity, but we will mention only three: face, content, and concurrent. Test-takers often have an opinion about tests; their perception of an examination is known as face validity. Content experts design tests; their expertise ensures the exam tests the material it is supposed to test (content validity). Finally, a test should correlate well with a previously validated test (measurement instrument) that was designed to measure the same thing; this is called concurrent validity.

> **Critical Comment:**   If you're beginning to lose patience and are sitting there thinking, "Just tell me what I need to know already, so I can do well on this test!" then whether you realize it yet or not, you need this book, so keep reading!

HOW ARE STANDARDIZED TESTS SCORED?

Initial scoring of an examination produces a "raw score," which is simply the number of correctly answered questions. The *percent* correct score is obtained by dividing the number of correct responses by the number of total items on the examination. For example, if there were 150 items on the exam and you answered 114 correctly, your raw score would be 114 and your percent correct score would be 76% (114/150).

Is the interpretation of standardized test scores so simple? In a word, *No*! Two practices make the interpretation of standardized test scores more challenging—the inclusion of pilot items and normalization of scores.

Pilot Items

Pilot items are test questions that do not count in the determination of your final score. Standardized test questions go through an item validation process prior to their use in determining an actual test score (Shrock & Coscarelli, 2000). This is to eliminate invalid and/or unreliable questions. To validate a question, it is included on an actual examination to see how it performs in a real-world testing situation—how many examinees select the correct answer, how many examinees select incorrect responses and which ones, did examinees from different areas of the country perform the same, and so on. This process, known as psychometric validation, uses a lot of statistics. The good news for you is that you don't need to understand how it's done; just being aware that it occurs is enough.

HOW DO PILOT ITEMS IMPACT YOUR FINAL REPORTED SCORE?

Your reported score (i.e., the final score you receive from the testing agency) reflects the number of correctly answered *scored* items, not inclusive of the pilot items. To better understand what this means, let's look at a specific example:

For an examination with 150 total items, 30 of which are pilot items, your reported score will be based on the number of questions you answered correctly from the 120 *scored* items, not the entire pool of 150 items. So let's say you answered 90 items correctly out of the total number of 150; what will be your reported score? That depends. It depends on how many of the questions that you answered correctly were scored items because your reported score is based only on the number correct of the 120 *scored* items. If, of your 90 correct answers, only 60 of them were among the 120 scored items, your final reported raw score would be 60 and your reported *percent* correct would be 50% (60/120) not 60% (90/150). What if all 90 questions that you answered correctly were scored items? Then, your reported raw score would be 90 and your reported percent score would be 75% (90/120).

So you can see that the number of pilot items on an exam can significantly affect your final reported score. Pilot items can also impact your *perception* of how you're doing on an exam *while* you are taking it. For example, during a standardized test, you might come across questions that seem poorly worded, extra confusing, or otherwise unexpected. It is certainly possible these represent pilot items. In order to avoid becoming unduly overwhelmed, worried, and anxious or distracted by these questions, we suggest you assume they *are* pilot items and will not be scored. Move on to the next question with no worries! We will revisit this idea in Section IV.

Executing Your Game Plan (Test Day)

To add another layer of complexity, on most standardized tests, your final reported score is not a percent correct score; it is a *normalized score.* Generally, the next question we are asked is, "What is a normalized score?"

Normalized Test Scores

To allow test scores to be interpreted in more meaningful ways, test results are converted into data that allow the relative performance of examinees to be compared. This data is referred to as normative data and is generally described as either norm referenced or criterion referenced. Although we will first discuss norm referencing, you should be aware that many professional and licensing examinations have shifted toward a criterion-referenced framework to assess examinees' degree of competency (Shrock & Coscarelli, 2000).

One way to normalize a score is to take an examinee's raw score (the number of correct responses on the *scored* items) and compare it to the performance of the entire group of examinees that took the same (or psychometrically equivalent) test. This comparison results in a percentile rank. Percentile ranks range from a low of 1 to a high of 99. Percentile ranks provide more insight into the examinee's ability than the raw score alone. As an example, a percentile rank of 90 indicates that the examinee's score was higher than 90% of the scores obtained by the group. Earlier, we stated that answering 60 items correctly out of 120 scored items results in a percent correct of 50%. If fewer than one-fifth of all examinees scored above 50%, however, then the score of 50% would result in a percentile score of at least 80 or greater, which makes that score of 50% sound more appealing, doesn't it?

There's a problem with comparing examinees using the percentile ranking system; the percentile range will always be 1–99. What if everyone who took the test answered fewer than half the questions correctly? In a percentile ranking system, no matter how low the raw and percent scores are overall, the person who received the highest score is always going to have the highest percentile score and that will be at the 99th percentile. Because a percentile rank indicates only relative performance, we would know nothing about whether any or all of the test-takers possess a baseline (minimal) level of competency that would be required to perform an important activity, such as practicing medicine or nursing.

Criterion-referenced scoring offers an advantage to individuals who use test results to make judgments about competency. Instead of comparing examinees to one another, criterion-referenced scoring compares each examinee score to a predetermined standard, which defines a "mastery" level of knowledge. The "cut score" (i.e., the score that predetermines pass/fail) is established prior to administration of the test by a panel of content experts using—you guessed it—a series of psychometric exercises and statistical standards to ensure that the cut score is valid. If an examinee's score is above the cut score, the examinee passes. Using criterion-referenced scoring, it is possible that all examinees could pass (or fail) the examination. The advantage to the examinee of criterion-referenced testing is that the score they obtain, and need to achieve to pass the exam, is determined by comparing it to a predetermined level of proficiency rather than just other test-takers.

SUMMARY

This chapter described the basic elements of standardized tests and contrasted them to teacher-generated tests. Standardized exams test a larger domain of knowledge and breadth of skills; they are designed based on predetermined formats, delivered under specific conditions, and scored using psychometric standards.

We have presented this information for the simple reason that individuals struggle with standardized tests because (1) they have trained themselves to pass teacher-generated, not standardized, tests and (2) they don't realize that studying for standardized tests requires different study methods.

Before proceeding to Chapter 2, please reflect on the following questions:

- What was the primary take-away message for you from this chapter?
- What information will be the easiest for you to include in your exam preparation?

Be sure to complete the Chapter 1 Activity before starting to read Chapter 2.

CHAPTER 1 ACTIVITY

Becoming a Better Standardized Test-Taker

In Chapter 1—Standardized Tests—we stated that "there is no such thing as a poor standardized test-taker"; however, there are individuals that could prepare better for a standardized test. Use the following questions as a guideline and comment on how you will approach each of the situations listed to help you become a better test preparer.

Table	
1–1	**Activity 1**

a. When reading new material, what can I do to give it more meaning for me?

b. What characteristics differentiate teacher-generated from standardized tests?

c. What makes higher-level thinking questions more challenging?

d. What techniques do I use to prepare for teacher-generated tests?

e. What techniques will I use to prepare for my upcoming standardized test?

Chapter

2

Test-Wiseness

In our opinion, anyone that has ever uttered the sentence, "That was a tricky question," should have said, "I didn't understand what the question was asking," or "I apparently missed an important concept while I was studying for this test."

Students perceive test questions as being tricky for one of several reasons. It could be that the question was poorly written, rendering it confusing or potentially misleading. Although this might describe the occasional item on a teacher-generated test, it will not be true of the *scored* items on standardized tests (pilot items may be another story). Another reason is that the examinee possesses only a superficial understanding of the content when a deeper level of understanding is required to answer the question. A third reason could be that the examinee adequately understood the content but didn't appreciate the context in which the question was asked. Finally, the author of the question might have simply intended the question to be very challenging; in spite of student perception, difficult or otherwise complex questions are not "trick" questions.

HOW CAN YOU GIVE YOURSELF THE BEST POSSIBLE CHANCE TO ANSWER TOUGH TEST QUESTIONS?

As mentioned in Chapter 1, most students learn to pass teacher-generated tests using a few basic techniques. One of these is listening for clues from the teacher about what's going to be on the exam. Sitting in the classroom you've heard teachers say things like, "This would make a great test question," or "This is really important," or "This concept confuses people because . . . so don't let this happen to you."Most students have learned how to benefit from listening for such clues. They diligently write them down, draw a box around them, highlight them, or put exclamation points in the margins of their notes. For many, these clues are an important source of information when determining where to focus their efforts while studying. However, this technique doesn't work with standardized tests. You don't know the people who wrote the exam. It's up to you to discover what is important and what will likely be covered on a standardized test.

Seeking information has a positive impact on test scores. Examinees who understand the significance of determining the content and skills that will most likely be tested will typically allocate the time required to find the information. Examinees who use this information when planning their study time with *purpose* and *intent* are more effective learners and tend to be more efficient, too. Examinees who engage in such activities are *test-wise*, and they tend to be rewarded with higher test scores. In fact, practicing test-wiseness reportedly increases scores by up to 10 percent (Kuncel & Hezlett, 2007).

If you use the same study techniques to prepare for standardized examinations that you used for teacher-generated tests, your performance will probably not reflect your potential; you are not being test-wise.

WHAT IS TEST-WISENESS? HOW CAN YOU BECOME A TEST-WISE INDIVIDUAL?

The concept of test-wiseness was first introduced in the mid-twentieth century (Sarnacki, 1979), and has since undergone revision and refinement. Although there are a variety of descriptions including the following: the "capacity to use the characteristics and format of the test and/or the test-taking situation to receive a high score," (Milman, Bishop, & Ebel, 1965), for our purposes, we propose the following definitions to draw a distinction between the concepts of test-wiseness and test-taking skills:

Test-wiseness: skills and abilities, used *in preparation for* an examination, that tend to result in higher scores.

Test-taking skills: knowledge and techniques, used *while taking* an examination, that tend to result in higher scores.

Being test-wise offers a distinct headstart toward the acquisition and refinement of study strategies (discussed in Section III, *Practicing Your Skills*) that promote highly-effective test-taking skills (discussed in Section IV, *Executing Your Game Plan (Test Day)*).

Critical Comment: If you're reading this book, odds are you're either test-wise or desperate. Either way, there are things you can do to refine or develop your skills!

Test-wise individuals generally ask a lot of questions and spend a considerable amount of time seeking advice and gathering information. They recognize that the more they know about an exam, the better their ability to effectively prepare for it. Test-wise individuals tend to be skilled at gaining accurate insight into the key variables that help them plan their studying. Two of these variables are test format and test content.

Test Format

Test format refers to such things as the types of questions that will be encountered and the administrative aspects of the examination, such as the total number of questions, how much time is allocated for the entire exam, how that time is distributed, and the like. This type of information is often readily available; it's probably even on the Internet, and may be as simple as an Internet search and click away (see Appendix A). In order to ensure the accuracy of the information, it is best to refer to an official source for the specific exam in question, such as the testing agency's official Web site or information brochure (check with your university or college testing center or academic advising office). Some testing agencies and companies have very complete Web sites that include information about the exam, tutorials, and even practice tests.

Although there are a variety of test item types (e.g., multiple-choice questions, true–false questions, matching, short essay, long essay), because the majority of standardized exams use the multiple-choice question (MCQ) format, our focus in this book is helping you prepare for a MCQ exam. It is important to note that, in spite of our emphasis on preparing for multiple-choice exams, most of the skills and study techniques are transferrable to other types of exams. More detail about MCQs is presented in Section III, *Practicing Your Skills* (for information about essay questions see Appendix B).

Test Content

Perhaps you haven't considered the importance of knowing what the test format will be; however, it's our guess that you've thought a great deal about test content, and for good reason. How can you begin to prepare for an exam if you don't know what it will cover? Test content should be a focal point in the design of your initial study plan and ongoing study planning. Your study strategies, including allocation of effort and study time, should be guided by test content. The more information and insight you have regarding what content to expect on the test, the less likely you'll end up thinking, "I wasn't prepared for that question."

HOW CAN YOU FIND OUT WHAT WILL BE ON THE TEST?

There are four primary and reliable sources of information that can assist you in making more accurate predictions about what will covered on an examination: (1) what the instructor emphasizes in class, (2) the course syllabus, (3) the course learning objectives, and (4) the "test blueprint." You are probably already familiar with items 1–3 as they pertain directly to teacher-generated examinations; however, these sources are not applicable to standardized tests. So how can you find out what is most important to study for a test created by people you have never met? Before we answer that question by describing test blueprints in Chapter 3, we would like to mention one potentially *problematic* source of information about test content—others who have already taken the test. Having gotten that cautionary note out of our system, we now turn our discussion to test blueprints and how they can help you prepare for your upcoming test.

> **Critical Comment:** Best intentions aside, there are problems associated with asking other test-takers what was covered on the exam. The items on standardized tests are copyrighted. Sharing these items with others is a copyright infringement. There are penalties associated with breaching copyright laws—monetary fines, loss of certification, cancellation of scores, and/or damaged credibility. These are not sanctions you want to face.

SUMMARY

This chapter was brief, but its message is powerful and important. You need to learn as much as you can about the test. You need to know the content on which to focus and the test format you should expect. Knowing these things makes you test-wise and will allow you to become better prepared. Test blueprints are a resource that will take you a long way toward becoming test-wise. If becoming test-wise is a goal, then Chapter 3 will be very helpful to you.

Before proceeding to Chapter 3, please reflect on the following questions:

- What was the primary take-away message for you from this chapter?
- What information will be the easiest for you to include in your exam preparation?

Be sure to complete the Chapter 2 Activity before starting Chapter 3.

CHAPTER 2 ACTIVITY

Becoming a Higher-Scoring Test-Taker

In this chapter, we learned that tricky questions are really questions that an examinee didn't understand or misinterpreted. Test-wiseness helps examinees prepare for tests by gaining insight into the test's

format and characteristics. Using the following questions as a guideline, comment on how you will become more test-wise.

Table	
2-1	**Activity 1**

a. What helpful information did I find on the website for the test that I will be taking?

b. Is the test that I will be taking all multiple-choice questions?

c. What have other people told me about the test? Have I verified the information?

d. Does my school, college, or university provide resources that I should access?

e. How can the information from this chapter help improve my study plan?

3 Test Blueprints

HOW ARE TESTS CONSTRUCTED? WHY IS THIS INFORMATION IMPORTANT TO YOU?

The skilled craftspeople that built your house, residence hall, or apartment had a plan to direct their efforts. Construction plans, drawn by architects, are called blueprints. They contain the technical specifications and engineering details required to ensure the final structure meets the expectations of the designer in terms of size, shape, aesthetics, and structural integrity.

The individuals that constructed the examination you are preparing to take also worked from a blueprint. It directed their efforts to ensure the test they created is valid, reliable, and fair. Among other things, the blueprint ensures that the complete domain of knowledge the exam is intended to cover is adequately represented by the questions. To maximize score utility (distinguish high-performers from low performers), standardized tests tend to cover a wide breadth of content. Wouldn't it be helpful to narrow down the playing field and know what will be covered on the exam?

A test blueprint (a.k.a. assessment blueprint or table of specifications; see Table 3-1) is a carefully thought out template that outlines the content and skills to be covered on a test (Coderre, Woloschuk, & McLaughlin, 2009). Being aware

Table		
3-1	**Basic Test Blueprint**	
		Content
Skills		

of and knowing how to interpret test blueprints will allow you to use them to your full advantage, making you more effective, efficient, and focused while studying. The test blueprint is a valuable study resource, but it is one that is often overlooked, most likely because many examinees have never heard of them, or don't take the time to find or review them.

As indicated by the name, a test blueprint provides the technical specifications of an exam by delineating the domain knowledge or content that the examinee must master, as well as the proportion of the exam that will be allocated to each topic and skill. In a very basic example of a test blueprint (depicted in Table 3-2), the columns catalog the content (topics or concepts), and the rows indicate the skills that will be assessed. The cells give the proportion of items represented on the exam.

Most organizations that create standardized examinations publish their test blueprints for examinees to review (for a list of Web sites see Appendix A). Again, you should be able to find these on the official Web site or in an information brochure published by the testing agency.

Table					
3-2	**More Elaborate Blueprint for a Test for Healthcare Providers**				
	Heart Problems	**Lung Problems**	**Stomach Problems**	**Kidney Problems**	*Skills Totals*
Diagnosis	20%	12%	6%	4%	*42%*
Lab Interpretation	15%	10%	4%	2%	*31%*
Therapy	12%	9%	4%	2%	*27%*
Content Totals	*47%*	*31%*	*14%*	*8%*	***100%***

Your institution's academic advising office, learning resource center, or testing center may have this information readily available or could direct you to the appropriate source. Because test blueprints are periodically revised, you should verify you have a current version.

Taking the time to find, review, and reflect on how to use the information available in a test blueprint is very important to your initial study plan.

Test blueprints can help you do the following:

- Identify key areas on which to focus so that you use your time more efficiently.
- Avoid wasting time on areas that won't be covered on the exam or prevent you from spending too much time on areas that are not as heavily emphasized.
- Avoid the costly mistake of overlooking important areas of study.
- Reduce the likelihood that you will be surprised by something on exam day.

SECTION I SUMMARY AND NEXT STEPS

In Section I—*Understanding Your Opponent*—our intent was to provide you with a new, different, or broader perspective about exam preparation. We introduced the idea that preparing for standardized exams is analogous to preparing for a competitive sporting event. In keeping with this metaphor, this first section of the book described a process for "getting to know your opponent" (the test).

Standardized tests differ from teacher-generated tests in a number of ways, some of which make them more challenging. However, we firmly believe there is no such thing as a "poor standardized test-taker." We hope to persuade you that success or failure is all about preparation— understanding what you're up against, identifying your strengths and weaknesses, developing your skills, and making sure you can truly show what you know on test day. The variables that make a standardized test different *are things you can prepare for,* but to do so successfully, you need to become familiar with the basic concepts we presented in this section: standardized tests (Chapter 1), test-wiseness (Chapter 2), and test blueprints (Chapter 3).

The remaining three sections of Part I discuss how to improve your competence through improvements in your self-awareness, knowledge base, thinking skills, and capacity to perform. Section II—*Developing Your T.E.A.M.S.*—is largely focused on you, the test-taker. It is intended to help you understand the significant effect of your behaviors on test performance (aspects of T.E.A.M.S.—Time, Effort, Attitude, Motivation, and Selection). Section III—*Practicing Your Skills*—is specifically about studying for the exam through increased learning efficiency and effectiveness. Section IV—*Executing Your "Game Plan"*—focuses on enhancing your performance during the test based on your underlying competence; in short, being able to show what you really know.

Optimal performance on test day requires making a commitment to changing your study approach through purposeful planning and incremental behavioral steps. To increase your level of competence so that you can score high on the big exam requires a lot of work; it's not easy. If you believe otherwise, we have a lot more convincing to do.

Before proceeding to Chapter 4, please reflect on the following questions:

- What was the primary take-away message for you from this chapter?
- What information will be the easiest for you to include in your exam preparation?

Be sure to complete the Chapter 3 Activity before starting to read Chapter 4.

CHAPTER 3 ACTIVITY

Using Test Blueprints to Your Advantage

In Exercise 1—*Drafting Your Study Plan*—we asked you a series of questions to help you start thinking about how you would create your study plan. Question #3—"Which books, computer programs, study aids, etc., will I use to help me prepare?" may have been a bit challenging. Now that you have completed Chapter 3—*Test Blueprints*—we ask this question a second time and provide some additional items to help guide your planning.

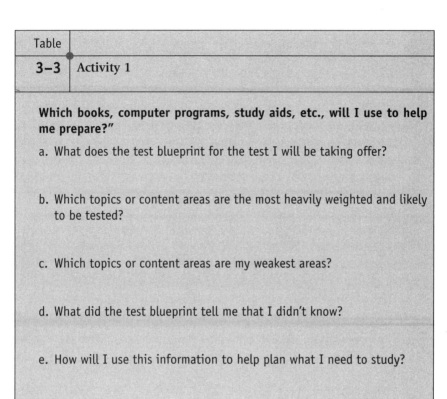

Table	
3–3	**Activity 1**

Which books, computer programs, study aids, etc., will I use to help me prepare?"

a. What does the test blueprint for the test I will be taking offer?

b. Which topics or content areas are the most heavily weighted and likely to be tested?

c. Which topics or content areas are my weakest areas?

d. What did the test blueprint tell me that I didn't know?

e. How will I use this information to help plan what I need to study?

II

Developing Your T.E.A.M.S.

IT'S NOT JUST ABOUT THE TEST; IT'S ABOUT YOU TOO!

In Section I—*Understanding Your Opponent*—we described the exam as a challenger you must become familiar with in order to optimize your preparation. However, you might actually face two opponents—the exam and *you*. Sometimes, we are our own greatest obstacles to achieving our potential. We contend that as part of your preparation process, you will benefit from thoughtful introspection and self-evaluation to get to know yourself better too.

In Section II—*Developing Your T.E.A.M.S.*—we will further develop the topics that we presented briefly in the introduction to the book. Obviously, as we are using it here, TEAMS is an acronym. Acronyms can be powerful mnemonics (memory aids) because they link a seemingly arbitrary collection of information with something more familiar, thus making recall easier. In this case, TEAMS highlights the important connection between the concepts of time, effort, attitude, motivation, and selection. Although TEAMS is useful as a rhetorical device, the sequence in which we will actually present the topics is MEA (Chapter 4), followed by S (Chapter 5), and lastly T (Chapter 6), but MEAST isn't nearly as easy to remember!

> **Critical Comment:**   When it comes to studying content, a topic in Section III—Practicing Your Skills, how you physically and mentally organize information while studying can make all the difference in the world. Sometimes you need to *reorganize* the information being presented to make it easier for *you* to remember.

Success in any endeavor is influenced by a variety of factors including, but certainly not limited to, your motivation, your beliefs about your abilities, your perception of your level of control over the outcome of your actions, your emotions, the resources and strategies you select, and how you use your time. Performing well on a high-stakes examination is no exception.

Chapter

4 Your Will

One meaning of the word "will" is the mental capacity to choose and initiate action (as in "will-power"). Humans act in purposeful ways; they are agents of their own fortune. We titled this chapter "Your Will" to emphasize that your exam preparation process, and ultimately your exam score, is largely the result of your choices and actions. Yet it is far more complicated than that because your choices and actions are influenced by a variety of factors, many of them relating to your psychology.

As stated in the introduction to Section II, Chapter 4 covers the topics of motivation, effort, and attitude. To ensure we're all starting on the same page, by motivation, we mean the reason behind the way you choose to approach a task; by effort, we mean a purposeful, determined attempt to accomplish a task or perform a behavior; and by attitude, we mean a way of thinking or feeling about a task/behavior. Because of their important relationships to motivation, effort, and attitude, we focus our discussion on three concepts: self-efficacy, locus of control, and academic emotions. Before we begin, here's a question for you to ponder:

Which of the following statements *most* accurately describes your beliefs about your exam score?

1. My score will reflect my intelligence and my problem-solving ability.
2. My score will depend on the difficulty of the questions.

3. My score will depend on what I do to prepare for the exam.

4. A high score will depend on my good fortune.

Think about your answer. We'll come back to this later in the chapter.

HUMAN AGENCY

Agency refers to the ability to carry out volitional (planned) behaviors—behaviors we consciously *choose* to perform, actions we *choose* to take, that is, they're controlled by our will—to effect change on the world in which we live. This is opposed to automatic (subconscious) behaviors, such as habits or biologically controlled behaviors (instincts).

Performance of a behavior (action), such as reading a book, requires (1) intention (will), (2) ability (personal characteristics), and (3) control. It is generally assumed that if you have the intention and the ability, then you will follow through with execution of the behavior. Whether or not the behavior achieves the desired outcome is dependent on the degree of control you have over the situation. You can intend to do something but not have the ability. You can have the ability but no intention. You can have the intention and ability but not be in control. Your perception of the level of control you have can also influence your intention; if you believe you have no control you are less likely to decide to act.

Imagine you have a strong desire to fly, unaided by any mechanical device. Can you do it? Now, imagine something a little less ridiculous: you want to swim in the ocean. You take swimming lessons and become very proficient. Can you now swim in the ocean? What if you live hundreds of miles from the nearest ocean and you have no means to get there? You have the will and the ability but no control over the situation. Now, to make it more complicated, what if, in the preceding scenario, your friend drives you to the ocean, but once there, you begin to doubt your ability to swim in the surf (after all, the pool did not have big waves)? What if you become fearful of being drawn out to sea by a riptide or being eaten by a shark? Will you be able to swim in the ocean? Will you choose to even try to swim in the ocean?

In short, there are many factors that either facilitate or hinder the process of human agency, and this, in essence, is what this chapter is about. The path from thinking about to actually doing something and obtaining a desired outcome is fraught with potential difficulty, and this might be your greatest challenge in preparing for a high-stakes exam.

In case you're the type of person who likes to know the conclusion before you read the whole story, here are three basic recommendations that flow from this chapter:

1. Believe you are capable of obtaining a high score.
2. Take responsibility for the outcome of the exam.
3. Develop and maintain a positive attitude.

If you would like to understand the rationale behind these recommendations, and we hope you do, please read on.

What motivates you to study for an exam?

A. Enjoyment of learning.
B. Fear of obtaining a low score.
C. Needing a good score to _____ (e.g., obtain admission to undergraduate, graduate or graduate-professional program; become licensed or certified).
D. Wanting to be the best.
E. Not sure.

Question: Why do we choose to do what we do?
Answer: Because we are compelled by our motivations to do so.

Motivation is the driving force—the incentive—that guides our volitional behaviors. Motivation is so important in achievement that differences in motivation have been shown to have a significant effect on differences in IQ (tests of intelligence) scores (Duckworth & Seligman, 2005). Motivation can be intrinsic or extrinsic in origin. Enjoyment, pleasure, and curiosity are intrinsic motivators; they are internal emotional states. In the multiple-choice question that we asked you to ponder previously, only option A represents an intrinsic motivator. In contrast, external motivations are rewards for performing a behavior, such as a specific object of ambition (status, money, career, recognition, or praise from others) or avoidance of an undesirable consequence of not performing a behavior (e.g., failure, rejection, ridicule). Your motivations for doing something might be both intrinsic and extrinsic. People who are primarily extrinsically motivated might not enjoy the things they tend to do; they do them because they want the reward. Consequently, when confronted with challenging circumstances, these individuals might find it hard to maintain a high level of effort.

Goals

Motivation has a reciprocal relationship with goals. On the one hand, motivation helps you achieve your goals by providing an incentive to maintain a high level of effort. On the other hand, having specific goals is motivating—it gives you direction and purpose; it gives you something to aim for. Football has an end zone, basketball has a basket, baseball has bases, and soccer and hockey have, well, a goal. Without specific, well-defined goals our behaviors tend to be rather aimless and haphazard. The literature is extensive on the positive effects of goal setting (Gerhardt & Luzadis, 2009; Kitsantas, 2002; Zimmerman & Pons, 1986).

In academic pursuits (e.g., taking courses or studying for a test) students tend toward one of two basic types of goals: learning-based (mastery) or performance-based (Ambrose, Bridges, Lovett, DiPietro, & Norman, 2010; Winne & Nesbit, 2010). Learning goals tend to be the objective of students who are intrinsically motivated by an enjoyment of learning or interest in the subject. They're curious; they aspire to expand their knowledge and are driven by a desire to improve their own competence. They compete against themselves, not others. Learning goals are associated with behavioral beliefs such as, "If I study enough and understand the material I know I can get an A rather than a B" and "The test was challenging, but I realize now what I didn't know and to be better prepared I will study a bit differently next time." Learning goals also tend to be associated with high self-efficacy and an internal locus of control, which we will discuss later in this chapter. Aligning your mindset with learning goals is a better approach to studying and more likely to motivate you to exert and maintain the extra effort required to be highly successful.

In contrast, performance goals are the objective of individuals who are extrinsically motivated to either be at the top or *not* be at the bottom. Performance goals are typically associated with behavioral beliefs such as "As long as I do better than everyone else, I'll be happy" or "I passed and that's all I needed to do." These individuals measure their success relative to how other people are doing. In our experience, students with performance goals do not typically enjoy learning or studying, they often become easily discouraged when they fail and they are much more likely to experience test anxiety.

We recommend you contemplate your driving force in taking and doing well on tests. If ultimately you cannot find it in yourself to derive joy, fulfillment, and pride from learning and developing your competence (and there's nothing wrong with you if you cannot), then give some thought to why you're doing this—it is, after all, your choice. Identify those reasons with which you have the strongest emotional connection, write them down, and put the list somewhere you will see it (e.g., on your bedside table, refrigerator door, or bathroom mirror) so you do not lose sight of why you're working so hard.

Developing learning goals (as opposed to performance goals) is not the only factor that influences motivation. Your beliefs about whether you are capable of doing what you need to do, your beliefs about your level of control over the outcome, and your feelings about what you have to do also impact motivation, level of effort, and performance.

RECOMMENDATION #1—BELIEVE YOU ARE CAPABLE OF OBTAINING A HIGH SCORE

Do you believe you have the ability to obtain a high score on your upcoming exam? If not, why not? What are you lacking? How can you obtain or develop the requisite knowledge or skills?

You probably have an opinion about your ability to be successful (or not) at various endeavors, such as driving a car or dancing. What's more, your estimation of your abilities probably depends, in part, on the specific conditions or parameters of the task, such as whether you have to drive in bad weather and high traffic versus on dry pavement with no other cars on the road. Similarly, you might know you are fully capable of shaking your hips to a beat in the privacy of your own bedroom, but have no confidence in your ability to dance an Irish jig in public.

Performance is far less dependent on level of ability than you might imagine. One major predictor of academic achievement is *believing* you are capable of performing the behaviors and actions necessary to produce a desired outcome (Boekaerts, 1997).

Psychologists refer to our beliefs about our own capabilities to accomplish a goal or perform a task as self-efficacy beliefs. Self-efficacy beliefs are complex, multidimensional, and contextual (i.e., they may vary depending on the specified parameters), as indicated in the foregoing examples (Kitsantas, 2002). Do not confuse self-efficacy with self-esteem. Self-esteem is perception of self-worth. You might have low self-efficacy for dancing an Irish jig because you know you lack the ability, but it does not affect your self-esteem because you don't believe it has any bearing on your value as a person. Academic achievement often impacts on perceived self-worth.

WHY IS IT USEFUL FOR YOU TO BE AWARE OF YOUR SELF-EFFICACY BELIEFS?

Your self-efficacy beliefs are important because they impact the goals you set for yourself, as well as the manner in which you approach tasks and challenges. If you believe you have the ability to perform well (i.e., high self-efficacy), you are likely to approach tasks as things to be mastered or achieved (learning goals). High self-efficacy is associated with increased effort and perseverance. In contrast, if you have low self-efficacy you might tend to avoid challenging tasks or situations because you believe you will not be successful.

With regard to test performance, you might have high self-efficacy for performing well on a specific course exam, but low self-efficacy for achieving a high score on a standardized test covering similar content. You might have high self-efficacy for each of the individual tasks required to pass a standardized test, such as reading, remembering facts, understanding concepts, problem solving, and filling in the correct bubble on an answer sheet, but low self-efficacy for sustaining a sufficient level of study effort over the length of time required to learn everything you need to learn. Obtaining a high score on a standardized test is not a behavior; it is a goal that requires the completion of a large number of intermediate tasks.

Let us now take a moment to remind you of a statement we made in Section I of this book: There is no such thing as a poor *standardized* test-taker. Doing well is a matter of identifying and developing the requisite skills necessary to become test-wise.

WHAT IS THE OPTIMAL LEVEL OF SELF-EFFICACY?

People with high self-efficacy tend to believe their success is related to their level of effort. They generally face obstacles as challenges to overcome and achieve high levels of academic performance. Yet, the dark side of high self-efficacy is "over-confidence." People who greatly overestimate their ability (have high self-efficacy even though they lack the necessary ability) often attempt tasks beyond their capability, resulting in failure and frustration. When individuals with overly high self-efficacy fail, they are inclined to externalize the cause and make the following types of excuses, "the test didn't cover what it should have," "the room was too noisy," or "the questions weren't written well."

In contrast, people who underestimate their ability (have low self-efficacy even though they are quite capable) tend to avoid challenging situations and therefore are less likely to improve their skills. These individuals often believe tasks will be more difficult than is actually the case. Failure is often internalized—"I'm not intelligent enough," whereas success may be externalized, "I got lucky." Low self-efficacy beliefs can lead to a reduction in the amount of planning and preparation, which increases the likelihood of failure and further reinforces the beliefs.

An "optimal" level of self-efficacy is one that encourages incremental growth and doesn't set you up for nearly certain failure, that is, a belief that you are slightly more capable than is actually true. This encourages you to set goals that will "stretch" your current skill set and allow you to be successful, with *effort*. Success tends to have a favorable impact both on self-efficacy as well as on motivation, especially when that success is perceived to relate directly to the amount of effort expended (Pekrun, Goetz, Titz, & Perry, 2002).

It is possible to alter your self-efficacy beliefs. We believe that the single best way is to experience success that is directly attributable to your own efforts. The following are some suggestions to help you begin the process of improving your self-efficacy:

1. Set incremental, achievable goals. Remembering the acronym "S.M.A.R.T." can help you learn to set good goals (Specific, Measurable, Achievable, Relevant, Time bound) that are just beyond your current skill level. This will increase the likelihood of your success and motivate you to exert more effort to set and then achieve even more challenging goals. In addition, as mentioned earlier, goals are a powerful motivator.

2. Become a self-regulated learner. Goals without plans are simply fantasies. Having a flexible plan, which involves breaking big goals into smaller subgoals, developing a timeline for their completion, self-monitoring your progress, and making necessary adjustments to your plan is more likely to lead to success.

3. Observe others who are successfully accomplishing the very things you wish to accomplish. Are they smarter than you are? Probably not, but they might have a better-developed set of skills, and this is something you can learn. (If you couldn't, we wouldn't have written this book.)

4. Seek friends, mentors, and advisors who will give you accurate, constructive feedback and positive reinforcement.

5. Don't mistake your fears and anxiety for inadequacy. Many highly successful, intelligent, skilled, and talented people experience fear and anxiety. For example, singer–actress Barbra Streisand has admitted to having such powerful "stage fright" she found it nearly impossible to do live performances. Emotional state is not always an accurate reflection of ability.

RECOMMENDATION #2—TAKE RESPONSIBILITY FOR THE OUTCOME OF THE EXAM

Do you frequently find yourself "hoping" or "wishing" for a high score? If so, you probably don't feel as though you have much control over your own destiny. In our discussion of self-efficacy, we mentioned several times the idea of internalizing or externalizing the causes of success or failure. We generally assign causes to one of two categories: internal factors or external factors. Internal factors are those related to self, such as innate abilities, personal characteristics, and behaviors. People who tend to believe their successes and failures result from internal factors are said to have an internal locus of control. In contrast, external factors come from outside of oneself, such as luck, fate, the actions of others, including supreme beings, and properties of the task itself, such as difficulty. Someone who tends to deny their role and responsibility in producing an outcome, and attributes causes to external factors, is said to have an external locus of control (Burns, 2008).

WHY SHOULD THE CONCEPT OF LOCUS OF CONTROL MATTER TO YOU?

Having an internal locus of control and therefore attributing the causes of your successes and failures to your own abilities, choices, and actions—sometimes called "owning it" or taking responsibility—is correlated with increased motivation, increased effort, high self-efficacy, and higher academic achievement (ibid.).

How we attribute causes to the events that happen in our lives affects our intentions (what we plan to do) and our actions (what we actually do), such as studying for an exam. There is more to it than whether a cause is due to an internal or external factor. Another piece of the puzzle is whether or not we perceive the factor to be under our volitional control. In the beginning of this chapter we asked you a multiple-choice question: Which of the following statements *most* accurately describes your beliefs about your exam score?

A. My score will reflect my intelligence and my problem-solving ability.
B. My score will depend on the difficulty of the questions.
C. My score will depend on what I do to prepare for the exam.
D. A high score will depend on my good fortune.

The question is really asking, to what do *you* attribute your success on the exam. What is your response? Each of the four options in the multiple-choice question represents either an internal or an external cause. Can you determine which is which?

Option A describes characteristics of the individual; option B is an intrinsic property of the exam resulting from the difficulty of the subject matter and the actions the person or persons who wrote the exam questions. Option C depicts actions undertaken by the self, and option D describes a supernatural force or coincidence of events, luck. Therefore, options A and C are clearly internal factors, and options B and D are clearly external factors. Which option, A or C, is most under volitional control? Which option is most likely to result in a greater investment in exam preparation behaviors?

As you are probably already thinking, when someone believes they have no control over an outcome, they are less likely to perform behaviors that could actually affect the result. When it comes to preparing for an exam, having an external locus of control implies that the amount of effort involved in setting goals, planning, selecting resources, and time spent studying is irrelevant to the outcome; ultimately the end result is due to factors beyond the individual's sphere of influence. Similarly, someone who believes a cause to be internal but beyond their control (e.g., because they are "a bad standardized test-taker") is also not likely to exert the necessary effort. Why bother, right?

One thing to keep in mind is that we often attribute causes on a relatively subconscious level. In other words, we don't necessarily consciously think about whether or not we caused something to happen. Similarly, how this attribution of cause affects our behavior is also likely to be subconscious; we might avoid doing something but not be able to explain why. Consequently, a person may not be aware of whether he or she has an internal or external locus of control. We don't recommend you spend an inordinate amount of mental energy trying to figure it out for yourself. Instead, just take to heart what we said in the introduction to this chapter; one way to improve your performance is to take responsibility for the outcome of the exam. Repeat this mantra: *How I do depends on what I did.*

RECOMMENDATION #3—DEVELOP AND MAINTAIN A POSITIVE ATTITUDE

Attitude refers to ways of thinking and feeling. We often make judgments about a person's attitude—"She has a *bad* attitude!"—and we recognize that attitude tends to impact behavior. We tend to do things we value and enjoy and avoid those things we think are worthless or find unpleasant. The emotions we feel, and indeed, our general mood (mood is a less intense but longer lasting emotional state), affect our intrinsic and extrinsic levels of motivation, our level of effort and persistence, our self-efficacy beliefs, the strategies we use, and ultimately our level of achievement. If you're happy and hopeful and take pride in yourself, you're much more likely to be motivated to work hard and long, and to believe in your own capabilities (Pekrun et al., 2002).

In terms of academics, the emotion that has received the most research attention is test anxiety; however, in spite of its extensive press and notoriety, anxiety is only one of several emotions that play a substantial role in academic performance, and in our experience is not the most detrimental to performance.

Emotions are categorized as either positive or negative. Positive emotions include joy, hope, pride, and relief. Negative emotions include anger, hopelessness, shame, anxiety, and boredom. On the whole, positive emotions, especially joy, hope, and pride, are correlated with improved academic performance (Pekrun et al., 2002). As discussed earlier, enjoyment of learning is an intrinsic motivation. It's not quite that simple, however. For example, although the negative emotions anxiety and shame tend to decrease intrinsic motivation, they can potentially improve performance through extrinsic motivation to avoid failure. Similarly, the positive emotions relief and contentment can reduce short-term motivation to study, leading to a reduced level of effort.

Research has demonstrated that emotions impact the learning strategies you use while studying (Pekrun et al., 2002). There is a correlation between positive emotions and the use of deep learning strategies and creative problem solving. Negative emotions lead to superficial learning strategies (e.g., rote memorization of details and rehearsal strategies) and algorithm-based problem solving. As you'll see in Section III—*Practicing Your Skills*—there's a place for both types of learning, but generally speaking, standardized exams test higher-order thinking skills, which are better acquired through deep rather than superficial learning strategies.

One negative emotion that shouldn't be overlooked is boredom—it is even more strongly correlated to reduced performance than anxiety (Pekrun et al., 2002). When you are bored you are, by definition, not intrinsically motivated. Furthermore, boredom draws your attention away from the task at hand (i.e., produces task-irrelevant thinking). When you're bored, you either mentally wander (i.e., daydream) or physically wander away from what you need to be doing. This is obviously not conducive to effective learning, and being bored with what you're learning can lead to procrastination—avoidance of what you should be doing. How to avoid these time-wasting traps will be discussed in Chapter 6—*Your Time*.

Even though test anxiety is not the only emotion that impacts academic achievement, in our experience, it's the one more students recognize as affecting their performance; therefore, it warrants greater attention. As we mentioned in the introduction, it is not uncommon for people to experience extreme anxiety at the mere thought of taking a comprehensive, standardized exam. Test anxiety can range from mildly annoying to profoundly debilitating. It can increase over time and worsen if the perceived consequences of failure are high. Test anxiety can impact not only exam day performance, but the entire process of preparation. Because test anxiety is reported to occur in approximately 25% of test-takers, it's likely you know exactly what we are talking about (Chapell, Blanding, Silverstein, & Gubi, 2005). It's important we begin to discuss it now and that you begin taking steps to manage it. If you suffer from profound test anxiety (you perceive that it has the potential to negatively impact your test score), developing effective coping mechanisms needs to be a part of your master study plan, right up there with selecting the right resources for your review.

Anxiety is a state of heightened arousal, an emotional, psychological, and physical response to a perceived threat. When you're anxious, your nervous system is activated, producing many physical and mental responses over which you have little conscious control. Anxiety (arousal) itself is not necessarily a bad thing. In fact, some level of arousal is required for consciousness, and a moderate level of anxiety is associated with increased performance. Anxiety about an upcoming exam, for example, can motivate you to study harder. Too much anxiety, however, has many known detrimental consequences, not the least of which is decreased performance.

Test anxiety describes excess concern about an upcoming examination. It can manifest both cognitively and physically. In a very profound way, test anxiety can affect the way you think—your mind can go completely blank or it can race all over the place with one distracting thought after another; you can have difficulty focusing on what you are reading; and you can have negative thoughts about not doing well on the test, perhaps even imagining that you will fail (Benjamin, McKeachie, Lin, & Holinger, 1981). Test anxiety can also affect the way you feel, physically—your heart can pound or race; your chest may hurt, and you may have difficulty breathing; your palms might get sweaty; you might feel nauseated or have abdominal cramps; you might get terrible dry mouth.

Most people recognize the physical symptoms of extreme anxiety or panic, but not as many realize the potentially negative cognitive consequences of anxiety, such as those mentioned previously, yet these can have an even more profound effect on performance. The physical signs can be distracting or even frightening, but anxiety-induced cognitive alterations get right to the heart of your ability to problem solve by competing with exam tasks for your brain's processing capacity (humans, like many first-generation electronic devices, cannot multitask). In addition, the symptoms of test anxiety can contribute to low self-efficacy beliefs.

Furthermore, while many who suffer from test anxiety know how it affects them during a test, they might not recognize how it can affect them prior to the test. For example, anxiety about an upcoming exam can keep you from studying. It can fuel procrastination. Procrastination can, in turn, increase the level of anxiety, often resulting in a downward spiral of discouragement, despair, and depression. The same kinds of negative thoughts that occur while taking an exam can also prevent you from adequately focusing on and learning the material you're trying to study.

In a very real way, test anxiety can impact you at every stage of the process, from the very beginning when you can't seem to get started, to the very end, when, after you've taken the exam, you replay the questions over and over again in your head, belittling yourself for every potential mistake. Test anxiety is so important that we gave it its own chapter (see Chapter 12).

Although excessive anxiety is usually emphasized as the major factor influencing test preparation and performance, a depressed mood state can also impact negatively on examination outcomes. Have you ever felt "down in the dumps" after earning a poor grade or thought "what's the use of studying" when preparing for an important examination? If so, you can probably thank a depressed mood for your thoughts.

A person's mood can be negatively affected by mental filters, which distort information and influence thinking processes. These mental filters are called depressogenic schemata. Schemata are stable cognitive patterns of thinking that serve as a template for organizing our thought processes. *Depressogenic* schemata are patterns of thinking that promote a depressed mood state, and they develop as a result of childhood disappointments and failures or from demeaning comments heard as child.

Once established, depressogenic schemata can lay dormant until triggered by a stressor tied to potential failure, such as a standardized exam (Sideridis, 2005). The most common depressogenic schemata develop around themes of rejection versus acceptance and failure versus success, both of which can relate directly to performance on important standardized tests. For an individual with a depressogenic schema, information related to the preparation and taking of a high impact standardized examination (such as that presented in this book) can become processed into a distorted sort of logic ("I cannot avoid failure" or "This examination is too difficult for me to pass") resulting from a depressed mood state.

Once triggered, depressogenic schemata promote a classic triad of thinking characterized by (1) a negative view of the self ("I don't have the study skills needed to pass this examination," "I am not smart enough to pass this exam," "I just can't focus on the material," (2) a negative view of the world ("These examinations are too tricky . . . or difficult . . . or unfair," "I should never have thought I could be a physician . . . lawyer . . . etc."); and (3) a negative view of the future ("Nothing I could ever do could make me successful"). This triad of negativity becomes an *automatic* (not under conscious control) way of thinking during times of significant psychosocial distress. The thoughts, however distorted, are adamantly believed to be true, and the resultant depressed mood state produces numerous negative consequences (feeling sad, dejected, worthless), behavior (low energy, withdrawal, lack of productivity), physiology (insomnia, loss of appetite), and cognition (pessimism, disinterest, loss of motivation).

"Surrendering" to the depressogenic schemata hampers the clear thinking required to adequately prepare for and successfully complete a standardized examination. To be a successful test-taker, under these circumstances, you must avoid surrendering to the distorted thinking and *take active steps to overcome your depressed mood state.* How? The best strategies involve expressing the negative feelings through talking or writing. Talk about your feelings with a friend, partner, or family member, and don't be inhibited by embarrassment or reluctance to reveal your personal concerns. Alternatively, you can write about your negative feelings in a *mood journal.* A mood journal is a concrete presentation of feelings that permits an objective review of your depressed mood state, making it possible to identify the distortions and patterns of thought that prevent you from focusing on preparing for the exam. Once expressed, work on replacing the negative feelings with positive feelings of confidence, security, competence, and an eagerness to take the standardized examination.

One of the recommendations we made in the beginning of this chapter was for you to develop and maintain a positive attitude, because positive emotions are so strongly correlated with academic success. What if you are bored with the material, dislike studying, are extremely anxious, and feel utterly hopeless? Are you doomed? No, of course not. Many people pass exams and obtain high scores while experiencing a negative emotional state. That being said, this book is about optimization—obtaining the best score you can, so getting your emotional house in order will certainly enhance your preparation and increase your likelihood of success.

SUMMARY

In Chapter 4, we discussed the relationships between motivation, effort and attitude, and behavior. We described how psychological concepts of self-efficacy, locus of control, and academic emotions can substantially influence your behavior and in so doing the outcome of your test (i.e., your score). Related to these concepts, we made three basic recommendations: (1) believe you are capable of obtaining a high score, (2) take responsibility for the outcome of the exam, and (3) develop and maintain a positive attitude.

If you are struggling with the ideas we've presented, if you have low self-efficacy, you feel as though you don't have control, or you experience predominantly negative emotions, there are people who can help you. Many educational institutions (high schools, colleges, and universities) have learning and counseling centers with trained professionals who can assist you in developing the types of reinforcing behaviors you need.

The remaining chapters in this section—Chapters 5 and 6—discuss the selection of resources (S) and time management (T), respectively. If we've done our job well, when you complete this section you will appreciate the significant relationship between these topics (TEAM**S**) and those we've discussed in this chapter (T**E**A**M**S).

Before proceeding to Chapter 5, please reflect on the following questions:

- What was the primary take-away message for you from this chapter?
- What information will be the easiest for you to include in your exam preparation?

Be sure to complete the Chapter 4 Activity before starting to read Chapter 5.

CHAPTER 4 ACTIVITY

Choices, Motivation, and Confidence

Chapter 4—*Your Will*—discussed the variables that affect our behavior. Keys to our behavior include options that are available to us and the actions we decide to take. Motivation and confidence are primary factors that determine our behaviors. The intent of the questions is to get you thinking about how and why you make choices. This insight should be used to help you plan corrective actions if necessary (Table 4-1).

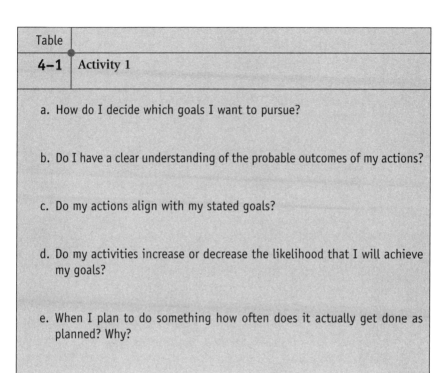

Table	
4–1	**Activity 1**

a. How do I decide which goals I want to pursue?

b. Do I have a clear understanding of the probable outcomes of my actions?

c. Do my actions align with my stated goals?

d. Do my activities increase or decrease the likelihood that I will achieve my goals?

e. When I plan to do something how often does it actually get done as planned? Why?

Chapter

5 Your Resources

As you prepare for your upcoming standardized exam, you will make many important choices about study resources. There are so many possibilities, how will you decide? Will you base your decision on the opinions of friends and acquaintances, or will you seek more empirical evidence and the counsel of experienced authorities?

This chapter focuses on two important decisions you will need to make. (1) What study aids you should obtain: standard textbook, review book, question-and-answer book, online test bank, flash cards, or prepared materials from a commercial review course? (2) How you will allocate your time to various study behaviors. How much time should you spend on techniques to improve your memory (retention and recall) of facts, answering practice questions, creating concept maps, tables, diagrams, and flow charts? What do you need to know about these various resources in order to make decisions that will bring you the greatest benefit?

The decision regarding which resources to spend your money on—textbooks, commercial study guides, and commercial review courses, especially those with hefty price tags—should be approached from a *caveat emptor* (buyer beware) perspective. Similarly, decisions on how best to use your study time should also be approached with caution. What study resources have been shown to produce the highest scores? What will give you the best return on your investment of money and time? The key is to make selections that will provide *you* the greatest benefit.

To set the direction and focus for this chapter, we first define and contrast three concepts: study resources, study aids, and study behaviors. *Study resources* are all the things you can use to maximize your preparation for, ultimately performance on, your examination. Study resources can be divided into two subcategories—*study aids* and *study behaviors*. Study aids are the physical materials you will study from. Study behaviors are the methods you will use to study. Individuals who routinely obtain higher scores on achievement tests tend to employ a wider array study behaviors than lower-scoring students. Furthermore, these higher-scoring students use their study behaviors more effectively and efficiently (Kitsantas, 2002). Higher-scoring students make purposeful decisions regarding how to spend their time. Although we introduce study resources in this chapter, the topic is so important that most of Section III—*Practicing Your Skills*—is dedicated to an in-depth discussion of study aids and study behaviors.

As we prepared this chapter, we reflected on the aphorism (look the word up if you don't know what it means), "Don't let the facts get in the way of your opinion." We find it troubling that hard-working students often spend a great deal of time, energy, and money on unproven resources and methods. In this chapter, we present to you the evidence. Ultimately, *you* will decide how to proceed. We hope you choose wisely.

Let's begin by reviewing factors that influence how decisions are made. How do your preferences influence your choices? How do your perceptions, beliefs, and biases cause you to make selections that are not optimal? The answers to these questions are dependent upon an understanding of who you are; self-awareness is a critical first step in understanding how you make decisions. A discussion of learning styles and learning preferences will provide some insight into characteristics of your personality that will ultimately help you make better, more informed decisions about your learning process.

PERSONALITY AND PREFERENCES AFFECT LEARNING

In the first paragraph of this chapter we asked the following question: Will you base your decision on the opinions of friends and acquaintances, or will you seek more empirical evidence and the counsel of experienced authorities? The tendency to make decisions based on subjective, personal assessments of friends and acquaintances versus using a more logical-analytical approach is strongly influenced by personality (Coffield, Moseley, Hall, & Ecclestone, 2004). Might the advice of a well-intentioned friend mislead you?

Personality traits—habitual patterns of thought, emotion, and behavior—including learning "style" or preferences, strongly influence how we study, how we process information, and how we make decisions. Perhaps the simplest definition of learning style is the manner in which you typically approach a learning task; however, just because you have a habit of studying in a certain way doesn't mean you have consciously selected the best method for you or for the material you're studying or that you can't (or shouldn't) do it any other way. Your learning style represents your "comfort zone"—the habit into which you will retreat when stressed—and it has probably helped you achieve some degree of success in the past.

Over 70 learning style classification schemes have been described, but the most common of them are characterized by the preferred method of receiving information through the senses—visual, formal text processing, auditory, and kinesthetic (Coffield, Moseley, Hall, & Ecclestone, 2004). Some people have one dominant learning style; others have more than one (i.e., they are multimodal).

Visual learners are drawn to images such as diagrams, graphs, and pictures, whereas formal text processors focus more on words and may prefer narratives, tables, and charts. Auditory learners prefer to hear information and may do well with audio presentations and live lectures, whereas kinesthetic learners prefer to use and manipulate information. People who prefer to write out their own notes and who enjoy hands-on learning experiences have a kinesthetic component to their learning style. Most of us can think of different circumstances in which we have used each of the four main learning styles. A preference is just that, a *preferred* way of doing something, not the only way of doing it. We can *choose* to do things in a nonpreferred manner, and in fact, the most effective learners are generally "flexible"—they select the best study resource for the task at hand. For example, if the learning task is to identify all the continents on an atlas of the world, they will study a map and use a visual learning modality. If the learning task is to be able to perform a mathematical calculation, they will practice doing calculations using a kinesthetic learning modality. If the task is to learn vocabulary words, they will use a verbal (written or auditory) modality.

It's best to match the study method to the material, rather than try to select a study method with which you are most familiar or comfortable.

Our personality largely dictates our preferences. Unfortunately, our preferences do not always lead us to make optimal decisions; sometimes our thinking is flawed or inaccurate. Our thoughts and decision-making processes can be skewed by biases we do not recognize or understand. What this means to you is that to improve your test performance, you should strive to become aware of your learning preferences and purposefully expand your ability. Selecting a study behavior that is not within your dominant learning style can be quite helpful and add significantly to your test scores.

Research has demonstrated that various aspects of personality are correlated with both learning preferences and test scores (Coffield et al., 2004; Sefcik, Prerost, & Arbet, 2009). Although a detailed discussion of this topic is beyond the scope of our book, we offer some insight into the impact of personality on test scores using the Myers–Briggs Type Indicator (MBTI) as an example.

Katherine Briggs and Isabel Myers developed the MBTI, which categorizes personalities into 16 different types by way of an extensive questionnaire (Myers, McCaulley, Quenk, & Hammer, 1998). The MBTI identifies preferences along four dichotomies: Extraversion-Introversion (E-I), Sensing-Intuition (S-N), Thinking-Feeling (T-F), and Judgment-Perception (J-P). Each of the 16 MBTI personality types is identified by a four-letter sequence, for example, INFJ or ESTP. The two letters in the middle (S or N and T or F) are referred to as the mental function pairs and describe how information is gathered (S or N) and how decisions are made (T or F). The S-N dichotomy describes a person's perception or awareness of their environment. Are they more in tune with facts and details (S) or possibilities and hunches (N)? The T-F dichotomy portrays a person's preference for making judgments. Are they objective and logical (T) or subjective and personal (F)? There are four mental function pairs: NF (intuitive-feeling), NT (intuitive-thinking), SF (sensing-feeling), and ST (sensing-thinking). Although no single type is better than any other type in an absolute sense, each type has associated strengths and challenges, depending on the circumstances.

As described above, the four MBTI mental function pairs describe how people prefer to receive information and then use this information to make decisions, such as selecting their answer on a multiple-choice exam. ST types tend to be analytical thinkers. They pay attention to details, are very organized and methodical in their thinking, and like to memorize facts. NF types, on the other hand, are abstract thinkers. They dislike routine and prefer creative, out-of-the-box problem solving. NF types intensely dislike memorizing and will go so far as to gloss over details, even important ones. NT types are big picture thinkers and try to identify patterns. They prefer to add details after they understand the big picture. SF types tend to learn best when they can relate (on a personal level) to what they are studying, and they tend to process information verbally. The fundamental, take-home message for you is that a preferred mental function pair has been shown to impact performance on different types of examinations, for example, aptitude and achievement tests (Sefcik, Prerost, & Arbet, 2009).

Aptitude tests predict future performance, whereas achievement tests assess past performance. Classic examples of aptitude tests are the ACT (American College Testing), SAT (Scholastic Aptitude Test or Scholastic Assessment Test), GRE (Graduate Records Exam), and MCAT (Medical College Admission Test); examples of achievement tests are the COMLEX (Comprehensive Osteopathic Medical Licensing Examination), NCLEX (National Council Licensure Examination), PANCE (Physician Assistant National Certifying Examination), and USMLE (United States Medical Licensing Examination). Research has reported that the mental function pairs correlate to scores on both aptitude and achievement tests (Myers et al, 1998). Intuition (N) impacts positively on performance for aptitude tests, whereas sensing (S) and thinking (T) impact positively on achievement tests (ibid.).

WHAT DOES THIS MEAN FOR YOU?

It means that regardless of your personality type (or learning style) it will benefit you to become flexible in your approach to studying. It is very likely that a partial explanation for the association between personality dimensions and certain kinds of tests is that certain approaches to studying are better suited to certain kinds of exams. All else being equal, the more closely your preferred methods "match" the exam requirements, the better you will tend to perform. Even if your preferences do not "match," you, as a human agent with strong self-efficacy and an internal locus of control, can choose to change what you do. If you are studying for a classroom test or a standardized achievement test (both assess what have you learned in the past), your score will likely be higher if you opt to study using techniques preferred by an ST type; as a group, these individuals typically score highest on achievement tests. On the other hand, if you're preparing for an aptitude test, studying using techniques that an intuitive (N) type would generally use could improve your score.

SELECTING YOUR BEST STUDY RESOURCES

Quantitative measures of studying are not enough. Through the years, we've repeatedly heard statements such as, "I memorized all my notes" and "I read all the assignments" and "I studied all weekend for this test." Simply memorizing factual information does not guarantee good test performance. Content is not enough. Studying for hours on end will not optimize your performance on test day. Time on task is not enough. *How* you choose to study is extremely important—quality matters.

Before diving into a discussion of study aids and study behaviors, we need to provide a framework. Ponder the question: what is the difference between studying to memorize content and studying to apply knowledge? Studying to remember content will generally enable you to recall information and recognize a correct answer to a question. There are study aids and study behaviors that can help you do this and do it well. On the other hand, studying to apply your knowledge is much more dependent on study behaviors than study aids. Students who perform well on achievement tests generally use a wider variety of more sophisticated study behaviors and use them in a more consistent and purposeful manner than students who achieve lower scores.

Study Aids

Study aids are tangible sources of information—*things* you can see, touch, and hear. Study aids allow you to review and rehearse specific content. The four primary types of study aids you will most likely choose from are traditional study aids, review texts, review courses, and question-and-answer resources.

Traditional Study Aids

We define traditional study aids as consolidated, condensed sources of information—tables, charts, figures, notes, flash cards—anything you can memorize. In Section III, we discuss these information sources in detail and provide recommendations on how to use them to maximize their value to you.

Review Books

Review materials with great (marketing) titles such as, "All you need to know about . . ." or "The easy guide to . . ." or "The only book you need for . . ." are often perceived as time-saving great buys. However, be leery of catchy titles that promise to make something easy for you. There is a lot of truth to the idea that if something is too easy, it offers little benefit.

Other questions you should consider when selecting a review book include: What are the author's credentials—does he or she have the background or experience to serve as an authority? Has accuracy and completeness been sacrificed for brevity? Will memorizing someone else's efforts at condensing, summarizing, and organizing the information deepen *your* understanding, or did it make the creator smarter? We are hopeful you will reflect on these questions, especially the last one, before making any purchases.

Having all the information distilled for you into easy-to-memorize packets of knowledge, although appealing, is probably not what you need. It might save you time but it's a short-sighted strategy and any short-term time gains will likely come back to haunt you when you're trying to answer higher-order exam questions. Where's your internal locus of control? What about self-regulation? To transform information into knowledge, you need to be an active participant in the preparation of your study aids; you need to create them.

Review Courses

If we told you that the result of over 20 years of research on the impact of review courses on exam performance suggests they do *not*, we repeat, **do not**, significantly increase test scores for the majority of individuals who take them, would you believe us? You should

(Kuncel & Hezlett, 2007; Sefcik & Obi, 2005). If we're not pulling your leg, then why do students spend hundreds of millions of dollars on review courses? We think it's because people believe review courses work and they're afraid that, if they don't attend, they will be disadvantaged by not attending.

Are there review courses that do benefit?
If so, what makes them different?

Effective coaching courses tend to share one feature. It's not the high fees, length of the course, amount of content covered, quality of the presenters, how long the company has existed, or even how great their materials are. Effective courses include lectures and exercises specifically designed to improve metacognition, test-wiseness, and test-taking skills (Bangert-Drowns, Kulik, & Kulik, 1983; Chaplin, 2007; Samson, 1985; Sefcik & Prerost, 2001). These things pay big dividends. Aren't you glad you are reading this book?

Question-and-Answer Resources

Question-and-answer (Q&A) resources are available for most standardized exams. They can and should be a major focus of your exam preparation process. In fact, as your test day approaches, we recommend you increasingly allocate more of your study time to completing practice questions. Q&A resources, in the form of books, software, or web-based services provide practice questions that are purported to be very similar to the actual test items. The computer-based formats can be particularly beneficial because many standardized exams are now themselves computer-based. It's good to practice answering questions in the same format as the exam. Furthermore, many of these computer-based resources have a "tutorial mode" that will walk you through the answer to the question, and most also allow you to create timed "practice exams," which is an excellent way to learn and practice.

As with other types of commercial study aids, we offer this cautionary note regarding the applicability of a Q&A resource to your upcoming exam: Who wrote the questions? Who wrote the explanations? What references did they use? How similar are they to the real exam in terms of content, style, and level of difficulty? Many of these resources claim to help you identify your weaknesses, but are they credible? Is there literature that supports their claims?

Fortunately, the key to using Q&A resources is not whether you have purchased the right book, software program, or online test bank. The key to Q&A resources is *how* you use them. We will discuss this more fully in Chapter 9—*Performance Enhancers*.

Study Behaviors

For our discussion, we have opted to use the following study behavior categories (Gurung, Weidert, & Jeske, 2010):

1. Thinking about the same thing in the same way,
2. Thinking about the same thing in different ways,
3. Managing your thinking, and
4. Thinking about your thinking.

Category #1

Thinking about the same thing in the same way is a study behavior called *rehearsal*. Although it is important to remember information, rote memorization—memorizing through repetition—is often inadequate for the task. It's fine for telephone numbers, grocery lists, and some classroom exams, but don't confuse memorizing with learning. Use of flash cards, recopying notes, or rereading a textbook chapter is rehearsing. When you simply memorize information, especially using a rote technique, given enough repetition, you will probably be able to recognize it, you might be able to freely recall it, but you will probably not be able to apply it. The types of test questions you are prepared to answer are low-level thinking questions—ones that simply require you to recognize and match facts to concepts, or that test your rudimentary understanding of a concept or principle. Just as an actor rehearses his or her lines for their role, rehearsal-based learning methods allow you to repeat exactly what you've memorized when you're given the proper cue. For an actor, the cue is usually another actor's line; for you, the cue is in the exam question.

> **Critical Comment:**   Preparing for a standardized test usually takes weeks, if not months. Therefore, it is in your best interest to retain information for the long term by moving beyond simply memorizing for short-term retention.

Category #2

Thinking about the same thing in different ways is a better study behavior that promotes real learning. A basic example is obtaining other people's perspectives. You can do this by studying with a friend, asking an instructor for help, or reading about the same subject in multiple sources, such as another textbook, a journal article, or a literary work. Using a rehearsal strategy, you might read the same thing three times; using this strategy, you would read three different things. Other study behaviors in this category include summarizing in your own words, drawing pictures, or creating concept maps. The chapters that follow describe these techniques and others in more detail.

Category #3

Managing your thinking plays a critical role in your success. Managing how much time you spend on various mental activities, including your emotions, is the foundation of this behavior. Do you (1) spend time worrying about what you should be doing or (2) planning your study schedule? Do you (1) spend time thinking about what others are doing or (2) focusing on your own activities? Do you (1) allocate most of your study time to rehearsal methods or (2) employ a variety of study techniques? Do you study (1) while listening to music with your cell phone nearby or (2) in a location purposefully chosen to minimize distractions? If you answered "1" to most of these questions, you are not maximizing your study potential because you're wasting valuable mental resources doing things you need not be doing. Although managing your thinking is important, it is not as important as the fourth category of study behaviors.

Category #4

Thinking about your thinking is a higher learning goal related to self-regulation. You need to get here. This mental behavior is referred to as *metacognition*. Cognition is defined as mental processes involved in acquiring knowledge through thought, experience, and sensory input. Metacognition is a level of brain activity above or beyond cognition; knowledge about how you acquire knowledge. Metacognition is generally described as self-knowledge about which learning strategies are most effective for a particular learning task or problem to be solved, and it's so important we've dedicated an entire chapter to it (Chapter 8). Self-regulated learning includes making plans (selecting strategies, developing timelines) to achieve your learning goals, monitoring your progress, and modifying your behavior to keep you on track. Self-regulation requires metacognition. Remember Einstein's famous quote, "Insanity is doing the same thing over and over again and expecting a different result." Don't allow yourself to become trapped in a repetitive pattern of ineffective study behaviors.

SUMMARY

As you prepare for the upcoming standardized exam you will be confronted with many choices, such as which study resources would provide you the most benefit. The decisions you make will be influenced to a large degree by your personality and your learning preferences; however, these "guides" do not always lead to optimal selections.

In this chapter, we attempted to help simplify your decisions by describing the different study aids and study behaviors you should choose from, and we offered some advice in terms of the kinds of questions you should ask yourself before you make any purchases or create your final study plan.

Before proceeding to Chapter 6, please reflect on the following questions:

- What was the primary take-away message for you from this chapter?
- What information will be the easiest for you to include in your exam preparation?

Be sure to complete the Chapter 5 Activity before starting to read Chapter 6.

CHAPTER 5 ACTIVITY

Selecting Resources

In Exercise 1—*Drafting Your Study Plan*—we asked you a series of questions to help you start thinking about how you would create your study plan. Now that you have completed Chapter 5—*Your Resources*—please answer questions #2 and 3 a second time. We provide some additional questions to help guide your responses (Table 5-1).

Table	
5–1	Activity 1

What study techniques will I use to prepare for this test? Which books, computer programs, study aids, etc., will I use to help me prepare?

a. What study aids would be most helpful to my test preparation?

b. What study behaviors would be most helpful to my test preparation?

c. How can knowing more about my learning preferences improve my studying?

d. Would taking a review course be helpful to me?

e. Which study techniques offer advantages over simple rehearsal or memorization?

Chapter

6 Your Time

Are you usually early or always late? Do you complete what you set out to do? Before you begin a project do you develop a plan with a timeline or dive right in? Are you easily overwhelmed? Do you have a hard time getting started? Do you avoid the things you have to do? Would your friends describe you as organized and inflexible or carefree and laid back?

In working with students, we have found that what might initially appear to be ineffective study methods is actually better characterized as poor time management behaviors. Unless you have unlimited time and resources, when preparing for an exam, any exam, you need to be *both* effective and efficient. Effectiveness refers to the ability to produce a desired outcome (e.g., using the right strategy to get the job done); this is the topic of Section III—*Practicing Your Skills*. Efficiency, on the other hand, is about maximizing productivity while minimizing use of resources (e.g., time, effort, money). The goal of time management is to become more efficient without becoming less effective.

Let's begin by changing the way you think about time management. People often have an aversion to the mere concept because they assume it requires leading an inflexible, regimented life and being enslaved by the clock and calendar. That's not what it's all about. For one thing, time management is as much about your attitude and values as it is about "management" and organizational skills. Time management is about figuring out what's important to you and what you want out of life, setting goals and determining what resources you need to achieve them, creating a plan to make it happen, and following through. Time management requires flexibility—the ability to adapt to changing circumstances—not rigidity. Time management can help you live a fulfilling life in a way that won't compromise your values and sacrifice your goals. You don't have to choose between enjoying your life and studying for your exam; there's time for both, but knowing when to postpone one for the other requires mindful planning.

In a sense, good time management is about having an internal locus of control (i.e., acknowledging that outcomes, such as getting to an appointment on time or preparing adequately for an exam, are a result of *your* choices and actions). For example, you might blame your tardiness on bad traffic or a train delay, but the ultimate reason you arrive late is that you didn't leave early enough. Some people are always early. How do they do it? They plan ahead and *anticipate* possibilities like traffic delays. Similarly, a low test score often reflects lack of adequate anticipation and preparation. Tardiness and low scores on tests tend to result from poor planning, poor execution, and poor time management (Chaplin, 2007).

HABITUAL VERSUS GOAL-DIRECTED BEHAVIORS

What comes to mind when you read the following: "Most of the time what we do is what we do most of the time. Sometimes we do something new" (Townsend & Bever, 2001, p. 2, cited in Wood & Neal, 2007, p. 843).

Apart from being a little circular, it's a reminder that we're creatures of habit. In fact, time management "skills" are largely habitual. We do what we do because we do it. Many behaviors related to time usage are automatic, triggered by environmental or mental cues—we go into autopilot and we stop thinking about it. To make matters worse, we often rationalize that what we do is *worthwhile* simply because it's what we do. We think, "this is important, otherwise I wouldn't do it."

There is a fundamental difference between habitual and goal-directed behavior, not the least is that habitual behavior is initiated at a subconscious level while goal-directed behavior is consciously controlled. There are even different brain regions involved (Wood & Neal, 2007).

A behavior may begin as goal directed but through time and repetition becomes habitual. Habits are beneficial in that they enable efficient, automatic action without the constant need to think everything through every time you do the same thing. However, this benefit of habits becomes problematic when the habitual behavior is bad for our health or well-being, or has become ineffective. Habits, good or bad, are notoriously hard to break or change.

We need to periodically recalibrate to ensure what we're doing really is important and worthwhile and aligned with our goals and values. We need to make sure we're doing the right things for the right reasons to get us where we want to go and lead us to the life we want to live. We need to reflect on why we spend valuable mental energy and time on things that aren't really important and that might in fact be self-defeating, such as waiting until the last minute to prepare for an important exam. Your attitudes, values, and goals are the foundation of effective time management and should guide your selection and use of time management tools and tactics.

TIME MANAGEMENT—THE TOOLS OF THE TRADE

There are many time management tools available; some are simple, like a clock, others are fairly complex. Tools are useful, even indispensable:

- If you don't naturally wake up on time, you set an alarm.
- If you don't know what time it is, you look at a clock.
- If you can't remember what you need to do, you make to-do lists.

Time management is not about tools, however. Owning a toolbox doesn't make you a carpenter. Deciding what to do, when to do it, and even how to do it is time management. Time management isn't even about managing time; how can you manage something you can't control? Time management is about managing yourself. It is a life philosophy, which when combined with tools, tactics, and strategies becomes a means of organizing your life and using the time you have efficiently and effectively.

This chapter focuses on the following five facets of time management: planning, prioritizing, scheduling, overcoming barriers to accomplishment, and maintaining a healthy balance.

PLANNING

●──

Before you create a "plan" you need to be aware of three important concepts:

1. A "plan" is only valid the moment it is created. You need to distinguish between plan, the noun, which is a static thing, and plan, the verb, which is an activity. We encourage you to engage in "planning" as an ongoing, dynamic process.
2. If you don't plan (verb) well, you'll experience false starts, frustrations, and increasing levels of anxiety, all of which tend to be distracting and counterproductive.
3. Most importantly, planning needs to be done by *you*, not someone else.

Planning involves a number of identifiable steps: (1) setting goals, (2) identifying the steps and resources needed to achieve the goal, (3) determining your priorities, (4) developing a timeline (schedule), and very importantly, (5) monitoring your progress and making the necessary adjustments to stay on target.

In Chapter 2 we defined test-wiseness as skills and abilities used by some examinees *in preparation for* an examination, which tend to result in higher scores. Test-wise individuals continually assess their progress. They tend to ask themselves, "Am I being effective? Am I approaching my goal?" and "What can I do to make improvements?" If they determine that their current activities (e.g., study methods or timeframe) are not moving them in the right direction—toward developing the appropriate skills and increasing their preparedness for the exam—they redirect their efforts. In other words, test-wise individuals are self-monitoring and adaptable; they are more self-regulating. Their plan does not lock them into a study sequence or protocol that doesn't work. They modify the plan as necessary to get them where they need to be. They are more or less constantly planning as they continue to gather and evaluate new information about their progress or lack thereof.

Begin with the End in Mind

Planning should be a mind*ful*, not a mindless, process—it's something you need to actively think about and attend to. A common error in the exam preparation process is starting without a sense of direction, without a goal, in essence, "winging it." Beginning to study without any plan at all often results in having to start over again (i.e., a false start), which wastes valuable time. However, if you tend to obsess over details, make sure you don't avoid starting because you want your plan to be perfect. For some, perfectionism and resultant procrastination can make it very difficult to begin. Remember, a good plan is adaptable, so don't be afraid to take the first step. We discuss procrastination later in this chapter in the segment called *Overcoming Barriers to Accomplishment*.

In Chapter 4 we talked about the relationship between goals, motivation, and academic achievement. Goals give us something to aim for and provide a standard against which to measure our progress. Setting specific, measurable, achievable, relevant, time-bound (SMART) goals is fundamentally important to time management. Goals don't have to be lofty—getting to an appointment on time is a small but SMART goal. However, big goals are also important because they give our life direction. These should be written down—to make them "real"—and shared with other people—to make you more accountable and to give others the chance to support and encourage you. We recommend you begin by making a list of your long-term goals and short-term goals in the areas of education, career, and personal life. How might your score on your upcoming test fit in with your goals?

As we've touched on a number of times already, having a goal does not mean you will achieve it; goals without plans are mere fantasies. Behaviorally, planning is one of the most important actions you'll perform in the exam preparation process.

Plan for the Worst

In Chapter 4 we discussed the benefits of having a positive attitude, and although we want you to be hopeful, we do not want your plan to be based on nothing more than wishful thinking. Therefore, in planning we recommend you adopt a slightly pessimistic approach. It is great to hope that everything will work out perfectly, but it can be detrimental to *expect* it always will. As the saying goes, "Life is what happens when you're busy making other plans." One important aspect of planning is being proactive, not reactive—anticipating potential obstacles and planning for the unexpected. How can you plan for something that is essentially a surprise? Good question. The answer is easier than you might imagine—be flexible. Identify alternative "routes," build in time "buffers" and "safety nets." Just as when you're creating a household budget—allocating money for rent, food, utilities, entertainment, and student loans—you might include a "miscellaneous" category or emergency fund, and the same principle works in planning and scheduling too. Make sure your plan can adapt to obstacles and surprises—build them into your timeline—and of course, monitor your progress and make adjustments.

PRIORITIZING

Life is messy and complicated. We rarely have the luxury to focus on only one thing at a time—from an early age, we begin to juggle multiple responsibilities and interests. It is a rare student who is not trying to balance school, work, extracurricular activities, family, friends, and numerous other opportunities and challenges. It is far too easy to become overwhelmed and lose sight of what is important. To be efficient and effective, you have to think about how you determine what to do and when to do it. Prioritizing—determining the order in which to do things based on relative importance—is an essential component of time management.

> **Critical Comment:** Everyone has the same amount of time in an hour, a day, etc. The difference in effectiveness is not based on the fact that one person has more time; the difference is based on how the time is allocated and used.

As we've said many, many times, planning what you *need* to do is critical to achieving your goals. We repeat—what you *need* to do. What you need is frequently not the same as what you *want* or *prefer*. Need is largely dictated by circumstances, including the goals we set for ourselves, whereas want and preference are often controlled by our personality (see also Chapter 5 for a discussion of personality). A reasonable exam preparation plan will inevitably include doing things you really, *really* don't want to do. It will entail self-denial, that is, not doing things you enjoy but that waste your time, and saying "no" to otherwise great opportunities because they will distract you from the important task at hand. It will entail delaying gratification. You might need to rethink your other obligations, and ask yourself some hard questions about what you really should be doing. In short, we want you to avoid common planning pitfalls, such as gravitating toward your wants (preferences and likes) as opposed to your "needs" or must-dos. You might want to study biology, but you <u>must</u> study biochemistry. You might want to go out with your friends, but what you really *must* do is get a good night's sleep so you're fresh in the morning. Your study plan has to be grounded in a process that maximizes the probability you will achieve the desired outcome (i.e., the highest score you can obtain). There should be nothing in your plan that does not move you closer to your goals.

Everything but the Kitchen Sink

In order to add "preparing for a standardized exam" to your already full schedule, there are two questions you really need to answer: *What else do I have on my plate during the time period in which I will be studying for my exam?* and *How much time do I have to spare?*

To answer the first question, we recommend you make a complete list of all your projects and tasks, with due dates. This list should include everything academic (write a paper, prepare for exam), personal (plan a birthday party, volunteer at homeless shelter), and job related (apply for lab teaching assistant position)—don't leave anything off. If you're taking classes currently, you might consider listing each course as a separate project.

Once your list is completed, cross off every item that is not important, not urgent, or not promised (at a minimum, move them to an "if and only if you have time" list until after your exam is over)—this is no time for "wish lists." Keep in mind the distinction between importance and urgency—they are *not* the same thing; important things are not necessarily urgent. Important things are beneficial—they fulfill a basic need for food, shelter, or health; they help us grow personally, intellectually, or spiritually; they enable us to achieve our goals. Urgency, on the other hand, refers to timeframe; urgent things need to be done now, not later. Something can be important and urgent, such as paying a bill or going to the doctor when you're sick, and something can be urgent, but not at all important, such as answering a phone call or attending a party. Things can even be important but not urgent, such as studying, planning, learning a new skill, spending quality time with your loved ones, exercise, or developing a hobby. Ideally, most of the items on your list will be important. With proper planning, very few, if any, items should be urgent. If possible, rank the remaining items on your list in order of their importance to you (or how dire the consequences if not completed).

Some of the items on your list might be simple one-step tasks, but, more likely, most of them are better described as projects, undertakings composed of several individual tasks. Before you can move on to scheduling, you should break down each of your projects into a series of actionable steps. Your ultimate goal is to identify the "next action" required to move the project along. These "next actions" will form the basis of daily to-do lists or will be included in your weekly schedule. The idea behind next actions is that people are much more likely to accomplish a task if it is specific and manageable. To illustrate the point: Which of the following are you more likely to do: (1) plan a wedding or (2) call the caterer? Which of these possibilities are you more likely to do: (1) write a term paper or (2) use a search engine to find ten articles on test anxiety? Get the picture? (In case you're wondering, most people would select "2.")

To answer the second question—how much time do I have to spare?—we recommend that you try to estimate how much time you spend engaged in various tasks and activities—from grooming to socializing—in order to gain a clearer picture of how you currently use your time (Time Utilization Exercise, see Figure 6-1). We have found that many people do not have a good sense of how they occupy themselves on a routine basis, yet this level of awareness is essential to good time management and effective scheduling.

SCHEDULING

Before you create your study schedule, there's still one more step—establishing a timeline. Scheduling is a process of assigning a time slot to your various tasks, appointments, and activities; therefore, you need to determine a realistic timeframe for your exam preparation, ideally one with a series of intermediate deadlines (short-term goals). In doing this, you will need to gather some information and make some decisions: (1) When is the exam offered? (2) How many days/

Figure 6-1

Time Utilization Exercise

Activity	Hours per day	Multiply	Hours per week
Hours per night of **sleep**.		× 7	
Hours per day **grooming/bathroom activities**.		× 7	
Hours per day for **meals/snacks (including preparation time)**.		× 7	
Hours per day of **travel/commute time** (Mon - Fri).		× 5	
Hours per day of **travel/commute time** (Sat & Sun).		× 2	
Hours **per week** for **scheduled activities including work (excluding** classes).	→→→→	→→→→	
Hours **per week** ACTUALLY spent in **class** (lectures and labs).	→→→→	→→→→	
Hours **per week** for **chores, exercise, errands, etc**.	→→→→	→→→→	
Hours **per week** for **socializing** (dates, recreation, movies, etc.).	→→→→	→→→→	
TOTAL (T) hours per week	→→→→	→→→→	T =

weeks/months do you feel you need to prepare, based on the study aids you need to review, the skills you need to develop, and the level of knowledge you currently possess? (3) What else will you be doing during this time period? Once that's accomplished, scheduling is a lot like packing a suitcase—you know how big it is (how much time you have until your test), you know how much stuff you need to bring (all the things you have to do and learn)—now, you just need to make it all fit.

HOW MUCH TIME SHOULD YOU SPEND STUDYING FOR AN EXAM?

Achieving the best outcome (highest score) is the ultimate goal for most. Nevertheless, some unknowingly sacrifice important elements of performance when preparing for examinations. For more than 20 years, the literature has reported that *total study time is only weakly correlated* with higher grades (Dickinson & O'Connell, 1990; Gurung, 2005). In contrast, the amount of time spent reviewing, organizing information, integrating concepts, and practicing what you'll be expected to do on the exam—answer questions—is a much better score predictor. It's the old (and often true) argument, "it's the quality not the quantity that counts." An optimal study schedule will specify periods of time allotted to different types of learning activities, such as reading a review text, answering practice questions, or creating concept maps (see Section III for a discussion of types of learning activities).

The problem with the question, "How much time should you spend studying for an exam?" is that there is no one-size-fits-all correct answer. It all depends—you should spend as much time as you need, and that depends on your starting point, which is exactly why you need to *know your* strengths and weaknesses, *you* need to set goals, *you* need to plan, *you* need to monitor your progress, and *you* need to be flexible.

Use an informed common sense approach to setting study-time goals. Get to know yourself well. Consider all the variables involved in making a decision. For example, most people have a sense for how quickly they can read text on a page—if not, then time yourself. If you know it takes you about 2 minutes to read a page, then you know you can't possibly read 60 pages an hour, right? So, don't schedule yourself to read a 300-page book in one afternoon. You are also probably intuitively aware that the amount of time it takes to read something depends on *what* you're reading and *why* you're reading it. Generally speaking, it takes less time to read the same number of words in a novel than it does in a textbook. The more difficult the material and the more you need to actively think about, mentally organize, and remember the information, the more time you need to read (and process), *so plan accordingly.*

A useful way to begin the scheduling process is to prioritize the topics you need to study. Use a test blueprint (see Chapter 3) to determine what is emphasized on the exam you are preparing to take and compare that to your strengths and weaknesses to determine what areas you most need to focus on to improve. Based on our experience, individuals who allocate *more time* to subjects they know *least well* dramatically increase their test scores. Many people do just the opposite—they spend the most time on their favorite subjects, which are often their best subjects. Why? Because it feels much better to study stuff we know and like. Generally speaking, it is best to begin with your weakest (and often least favorite) topics. That way, as you progress through the preparation process and your energy level inevitably drops, the material you're reviewing becomes easier and more engaging, instead of harder and less appealing. Unfortunately, it has been our experience that far too many individuals either do not create a study timeline based on the principle of need or create an underdeveloped timeline, lacking necessary detail and direction.

WHAT SHOULD MY STUDY SCHEDULE LOOK LIKE?

In its most rudimentary form a study schedule is essentially a grid or matrix of content (what you need to study) and time (when you will do it) (see Figure 6-2). A filled-out weekly calendar can suffice, but creating a custom grid using a spreadsheet or word processing program allows you greater flexibility. The grid can be further divided to include details of what will be studied (topics and learning goals), what resources will be used (notes, books, or question banks) on which days and for how long (see Figure 6-3). Your entire schedule may span a week, a few weeks, or a few months; it all depends on when you are taking your exam, when you will begin studying, and how much you need to cover. There are many possible ways to design a study schedule. Using your favorite search engine, surf the Internet for "study schedule" and see what you find. You can probably locate a template that is appealing to you, but don't simply use someone else's study

Figure 6-2

Basic Study Schedule

	Monday	Tuesday	Wednesday	Thursday	Friday	Saturday	Sunday
Week 1	Topic A	Topic B	Topic C	Topic D	Topic C	OFF	Topic D
Week 2	Topic B	Topic E	Topic B	Topic F	Topic C	Topic A	OFF
Week 3	Topic C	Topic E	Topic B	OFF	Topic F	Topic C	Topic D
Week 4	Topic B	OFF	Topic A	Topic F	Topic C	Topic E	OFF

Figure 6-3

Detailed Study Schedule

Study Day	Date	Topic/Task	Details/Learning Goals	Resources	Est. Time
1					
2					
3					
4					
5					
6					
7					
8					
9					
10					
...					
...					
...					
42					

schedule—you should always customize whatever you find to suit your unique circumstances and needs.

Developing a Master Schedule

It might seem like a lot of extra work, but for maximal organization, we recommend you develop two different types of schedules. One schedule will be a detailed study schedule/plan for your exam preparation that specifies what activities you will accomplish on what days (Figure 6-3). The other (a master schedule) will include, in a less detailed way, *everything* you need to do (all your projects, tasks,

Figure 6-4

Weekly "Master" Schedule

Time	Monday	Tuesday	Wednesday	Thursday	Friday	Saturday	Sunday
6am	Coffee/ Bagel	Coffee/ Yogurt	Coffee/ Bagel	Coffee/ Muffin	Coffee/ Cereal	Sleep	Sleep
7	Preview lectures	Preview & Review	Preview & Review	Preview & Review	Preview & Review	Coffee	Coffee & Weekly schedule review
8							
9	Lectures	Lectures	Lectures	Lectures	Lectures	Chores	Personal growth/ reflection
10							
11							
12	Lunch	Lunch	Lunch	Lunch	Lunch	Lunch	Lunch
1pm	Lab	Something fun!	Preview Lab Materials	Study	Study	Study	Chores
2							
3		Study	Lab				
4							
5	Exercise	Exercise	Exercise	Exercise	Exercise	Exercise	Exercise
6	Dinner	Dinner	Dinner	Dinner	Dinner	Dinner	Dinner
7	Personal/ Family time	Personal/ Family time	Personal/ Family time	Personal/ Family time	Recreation/ Socializing	Recreation/ Socializing	Study
8	Study	Study	Study	Study			
9							
10							
11	Sleep	Sleep	Sleep	Sleep			Sleep

chores, appointments, recreational activities, etc.) (Figure 6-4). This "master schedule" will ensure you don't lose sight of anything during this important, but potentially hectic, period of time. You could try to consolidate your detailed study plan and your weekly calendar into one document; however, it will likely become overly cluttered and hard to follow, hence overwhelming, which will defeat the purpose. You want to be organized and in control but not give yourself something else to worry about.

When filling in your study schedule, keep these general principles in mind:

- Studying is most effective when spread out over a longer period of time, a concept known as distributed effort or spaced studying (Medina, 2008). This is the opposite of cramming (McIntyre & Munson, 2008).
- You need to be realistic. As mentioned before, don't schedule more than you can actually accomplish or you may become frustrated, discouraged, and anxious.
- You need to be flexible. Things come up that you don't expect—that's life. Build flexibility into your schedule either by allowing one day each week to be an overflow day, or simply by not scheduling every minute of every day for studying.
- Review your schedule at least once a week and revise as needed.
- Keep in mind all the other things you have to do in your life. While you're preparing for the exam, you may want to create a master schedule that includes everything you need to do (all obligations, projects, activities).
- Schedule pleasurable activities as well as obligations. By putting them in a different color (or using a different font), they stand out and give you something to look forward to.
- The more specific your calendar entries, the more likely you will actually follow through with them (remember your "next actions").

Schedules versus To-Do Lists

Daily to-do lists can be very helpful and motivating, but they are not a substitute for a detailed schedule. Ideally, your weekly master schedule will *include* predictable errands and chores, with an assigned day and time; for example, Wednesday 3–4 pm is grocery shopping, Saturday 9 am–12 pm is house cleaning, and Monday 8–10 pm is laundry. Reserve your daily to-do lists for two types of activities: last minute or unexpected tasks and appointments and "next actions" for your main projects. Each day, identify up to five items for your to-do list. Scattered throughout most days are little snippets of time—10 minutes here, 15 minutes there—which often go unused. These bits of time can be very productive and used to accomplish tasks from your daily to-do list. Crossing items off your to-do list has the added benefit of providing a sense of accomplishment.

OVERCOMING BARRIERS TO ACCOMPLISHMENT

Unfortunately, even with a great plan, you can still fail to accomplish your goals. In order for something to get done, your plan has to be followed, which requires action on your part. Furthermore, although action is necessary, not all action is created equal. Sometimes, for the sake of "doing more," we try to do many things simultaneously, which, as we shall argue, is not efficient or effective. In discussing time management, we would be remiss if we didn't address two major barriers to getting things done—procrastination and multitasking.

Procrastination

Procrastination refers to behaviors that needlessly postpone actions or tasks to a later time, often resulting in negative personal consequences (e.g., obtaining poor grades, earning a reputation as a slacker, feeling guilty or anxious). Procrastination can be absolutely debilitating to the exam preparation process, not to mention overall quality of life. Procrastination might be limited to a very specific task or circumstance, or it might represent a long-term pattern of behavior, perhaps something you've done for years. If you tend to procrastinate, is your avoidance behavior associated always with school, with a specific course, a specific type of task (e.g., writing or studying for an exam), only when you're not interested in the task, or do you procrastinate whenever there is something you should be doing?

Procrastination is *extremely* common among students, and its causes are many, including:

- Boredom/apathy
- Feeling overwhelmed by the magnitude of a task
- Feeling overwhelmed by the number of tasks

- Perfectionism
- Fear of failure
- Pressures of success
- Resentment toward the task or person making you do the task

Techniques to Overcome Procrastination

Regardless of why you procrastinate, avoidance behaviors can become a bad habit and overcoming procrastination takes time and effort. There are numerous techniques to help you minimize procrastination, but if none of these seem to work for you, we strongly encourage you to meet with an academic advisor or counselor at your educational institution.

1. Find or create a productive, distraction-free environment in which to work.
2. Break big projects into smaller "next action" steps. This is particularly useful if you procrastinate when overwhelmed or do not know how to begin.
3. Choose a task or step at random and complete it.
4. Put everything you need to complete the task right in front of you.
5. Set a timer for 10 minutes and promise yourself you'll work until it goes off.
6. Keep a reverse to-do list and write items down as you complete them.
7. Take a 10-minute break then try again. Set a timer so your 10-minute refresher does not turn into a much longer break.
8. Develop a reward system that incorporates delayed gratification—you don't get your reward until you've accomplished a step. Set aside some time each day to do something enjoyable *after* you've accomplished a study goal. Avoid negotiating with yourself by thinking things like "I'll go to the movie now and study when I get back."
9. Find a study partner, someone to help you get started and keep you on task.
10. Keep a journal of your thoughts and feelings about studying. Develop positive "self-talk." Challenge your negative assumptions about the difficulty of the task or your ability to perform a task. Tell yourself that you can and *will do it*.

11. Keep a time journal—every hour, write down what you did for that hour, including avoidance behaviors. What did you do instead of studying?
12. Reevaluate your goals and priorities. How does the task you're avoiding fit in with the bigger picture of your life?

The Myth of Multitasking

Our advice regarding multitasking is simple and straightforward—don't do it. (Actually, when it comes to cognitive activities, it's not possible, so stop trying.)

While you've been reading this book, have you checked your email, read or sent a text message, Tweeted, or Googled? Do you do these sorts of things while you are studying? If so, you're attempting to multitask. We say "attempting" because humans can't do it; instead, we switch task. Our brains move back and forth between tasks; we cannot do (or think about) more than one complex thing at one time. People might believe they are "good" multitaskers. They're not. People think so-called multitasking is saving them time; they think they're being efficient. They're not. Research clearly demonstrates that although we think we're getting more done, productivity actually declines when we try to do several things simultaneously. Every time your brain switches from one task to another, precious time is lost. The more switching that is done, the more time that gets lost (Medina, 2008; Rubinstein, Meyer, & Evans, 2001).

Have you ever been so distracted while you were talking that you used the wrong word? "The length of the hypotenuse of a right triangle is equal to the square root of the sum of the *hamburgers* of the other two sides." If we asked you to start counting ceiling tiles, and after a bit we started saying random numbers out loud, do you think you would lose your place? Distractions divide or divert your attention—they provide a novel stimulus that makes your brain "sit up and take notice." When your attention is drawn to something in the environment, that information enters your working memory and competes for processing with other information that is needed to perform some other task, such as avoiding a collision while driving, learning an important concept, or solving a problem (for more about memory, see Chapter 7).

Multitasking is one big distraction. The problem with multitasking while studying is that you're not fully mentally engaged in the important task: learning the material. Probably one of the reasons why people think they are capable of multitasking is that when they combine tasks requiring little thought, such as walking and chewing gum, it generally turns out OK. However, if you start to combine *more* cognitive tasks, like doing mental arithmetic and talking at the same time, it becomes more challenging, even impossible; thus, your effectiveness suffers.

The detrimental effect of multitasking on productivity and learning is backed up by abundant research. Research on multitasking demonstrates that distractions affect how memories are formed and that the knowledge obtained while distracted is less flexible—it cannot be transferred from one context to another (transfer, as an important part of deep learning, is discussed in Chapter 7). Furthermore, people who tend to multitask are much less able to filter out irrelevant information—they are more easily distracted and more likely to form erroneous memories. This is all bad news for learning and for future test scores (Ellis, Daniels, & Jauregui, 2010).

So, what can you do? You can manage your time so that you can focus on one thing at a time. If you have multiple projects or tasks all competing for your attention, schedule them sequentially. When you're studying, turn off your cell phone, stop texting, quit checking your email every few minutes, and turn off your audible notifications. Even listening to music can be counterproductive. If you can't study in silence, select music that will function as background noise that tends to "disappear," not something you want to actively listen to or sing along with.

The corporate world has begun to recognize the perils of multitasking for business executives; it's time you do as well. Once you've accepted that multitasking isn't possible, it becomes clearer what to do and, more importantly, what to avoid.

MAINTAINING A HEALTHY BALANCE

As we conclude this chapter on time management, we need to address a topic we have to this point neglected—maintaining a healthy balance. Adequate sleep, a healthy diet, regular exercise, and maintaining a social support network are actually quite important for cognition and learning, and quality of life. Although we cannot do ample justice to this topic, we mention it here because all too often, when students become fixated on exam performance, healthy behaviors are the first to go (assuming they were present in the first place; if not, then now is a good time to develop some). Generally speaking, most people accept that these things are important; the trick is making them a priority and finding the time to "fit" them in, which is why they're mentioned here, in a chapter on time management. We think these things are important enough to go on your master schedule, and the following guidelines will offer you a place to start.

Sleep

Adequate restful sleep is essential for learning, memory, and peak cognitive performance. Humans need an average of 7–9 hours of sleep *every* night; you are not an exception (Medina, 2008). The exact amount of sleep you need changes as you age and is affected by your health status and stress levels. If you are sick or stressed out, you'll need more sleep, even though being sick and stressed out will probably make it hard to sleep, a cruel irony of nature. How do you know if you're getting enough? As a general rule of thumb, if you feel relatively awake within 45 minutes of waking in the morning, you are probably getting enough sleep. If you find yourself dozing off during the day, you are probably sleep deprived. If you fall asleep in less than five minutes after you lay down, you are probably sleep deprived. It is particularly important to get enough sleep prior to taking an exam, but sleep deprivation at any time will impact negatively on cognitive performance and reduce the overall effectiveness and efficiency of your studying.

Diet

Rather than prescribing a specific diet that optimizes brain function, we will simply mention a few things to avoid: alcohol, excessive caffeine, and simple carbohydrates. For most people, the best diet for thinking is the best diet for health—low in fat and high in complex carbohydrates with an emphasis on a wide variety of minimally processed whole grains, vegetables, fruits, and low-fat protein (e.g., beans, lean meats, eggs). Your brain works best when it is adequately hydrated—dehydration can make you feel mentally sluggish and cause headaches—drinking fresh (unsweetened) water is a good way to accomplish this.

Although caffeine can boost cognitive performance, it is also habit forming and, because it has a long half-life in the body, can cause insomnia. That being said, for most people, a morning cup (8 ounces) of coffee is fine. Alcohol is a central nervous system depressant and, along with other potential negative social and health effects, it impairs cognition and can reduce the quality of your sleep. Although your brain requires glucose to function, your body breaks down complex molecules into glucose during digestion, so you don't need to eat simple carbohydrates. In terms of studying, foods sweetened with sugar, such as candy and soda pop, might give you an energy boost, but it will be short-lived and you will most likely crash...hard. In terms of time management, eating healthfully can require planning ahead. Convenience stores, fast food restaurants, and vending machines are notorious for having foods and beverages that are not particularly healthy. When creating your master schedule, make time for grocery shopping, food preparation, and sit-down meals.

Exercise

Regular aerobic exercise has numerous short-term and long-term mental and physical health benefits. It increases blood flow to the brain, boosts cognitive performance, improves the quality of sleep, reduces stress, anxiety, and depression, and enhances your mood. All these benefits can be obtained from just 15 minutes of aerobic exercise each day. You do not need a gym membership, fancy equipment, special clothes, or a lot of time. All you need to do is periodically get up from your books and take a hike around the building or climb a few flights of stairs. For a socializing bonus, take a brisk walk with a friend or study partner.

Support

Having a social support network is statistically correlated with a longer lifespan, but it has more immediate benefits as well (Shirom, Toker, Alkaly, Jacobson, & Balicer, 2011). Beyond having people—family, friends, peers, colleagues, mentors—with whom you can rest, relax, and converse, it's important to make the time to nurture healthy relationships for emotional and practical reasons. As we mentioned earlier, it's beneficial to share your goals and have someone to whom you're accountable. In Chapter 4, we talked about improving your self-efficacy through constructive feedback from people who know you and avoiding surrendering to distorted thinking resulting from depressogenic schemata by expressing your feelings to someone. Furthermore, you might need a favor some time—someone to give you a ride, take care of your pet or children, water your plants, watch your stuff, loan you a few bucks for a good meal, or any number of things. Having people in your life you care about and who care about you affords a type of safety net that cannot be acquired any other way. For all these reasons and more, include socializing in your master schedule. Thoughtful communication is among the most important factors in maintaining good relationships. Whether it's scheduling a phone call, a visit, a meal, a walk, or a study break, make sure you don't neglect the people in your life.

SUMMARY

Time management begins with attitude and ends with successful outcomes. Do you see time as a relevant factor in your exam preparation process, a resource you can use to your advantage, or is it something that works against you? Time management is much more than schedules and planners and to-do lists. To be good at time management requires managing your own behavior.

In this chapter we discussed setting goals, planning, prioritizing, and scheduling. We suggested not only creating a detailed study schedule, but also developing a master schedule that will allow you to incorporate studying for your standardized exam into your life in a way that doesn't compromise your mental and physical health or your relationships. We also pointed out that having goals and making plans does not guarantee follow through. You, as a thoughtful human agent, can either carry out your plans or sabotage yourself through your choices, such as procrastination and multitasking. You are the one who makes the choices, then follows through or not.

We hope this chapter has provided you with useful ideas and tools, which will ultimately lead to you achieving your highest score possible, but beyond that, we hope you will successfully incorporate time management practices into your everyday life.

SECTION II SUMMARY AND NEXT STEPS

The single most important message in Section II—*Developing Your TEAMS*—is that you are in control. You can decide, right now, if you will be sufficiently prepared for your test. Your attitude, your motivation, your effort, time you allocate to studying, and the selections you make with regard to your study resources all impact your test score. In the first section, we presented your opponent—the test. In this section, we offered advice on how to avoid becoming your second opponent.

There are things that you need to know; there are things that you should do as you prepare for your test. In Chapters 1–6, we introduced you to some factors about the test and yourself that you need to know and reflect on. In Section III—*Practicing Your Skills*—we delve more deeply into the types of actions you need to take as you prepare.

If you're tired, if now is not a good time, if you're pressed for time at the moment, if you're feeling unfocused—take a break, regroup, get some rest, reallocate your time . . . take control.

Before proceeding to Chapter 7, please reflect on the following questions:

- What was the primary take-away message for you from this chapter?
- What information will be the easiest for you to include in your exam preparation?

Be sure to complete the Chapter 6 Activity before starting to read Chapter 7.

Don't start the next section until you've rallied your TEAMS. When ready, return to the book and start Chapter 7.

CHAPTER 6 ACTIVITY

Time Management

In Chapter 6—*Your Time*—we brought to your attention that a major component of ineffective studying is not the techniques chosen but the allocation and management of time. The goal of time management is to become more efficient without becoming less effective. Answer the following questions to determine things you can do to become better at managing your time.

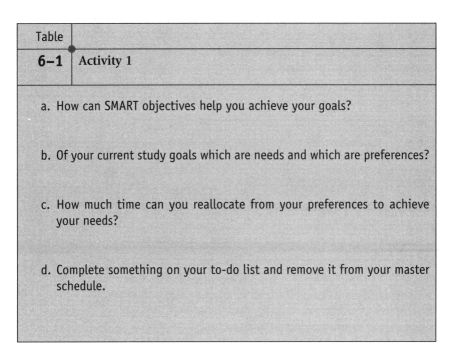

Table	
6–1	**Activity 1**

a. How can SMART objectives help you achieve your goals?

b. Of your current study goals which are needs and which are preferences?

c. How much time can you reallocate from your preferences to achieve your needs?

d. Complete something on your to-do list and remove it from your master schedule.

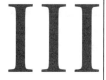

Section

III

Practicing Your Skills

High performers tend to share some traits. They have organized "mental filing systems." They are adept at recognizing patterns and relationships in information, which they use to help them remember facts and details. They are skilled at understanding what a question is asking and they have a reliable process for selecting the best answer. The people who achieve the highest scores on tests aren't necessarily the smartest people taking the test, but they are generally those who prepared the smartest way.

High performers know, at least on an intuitive level, the difference between a study behavior and study strategy. Based on the parameters of the exam, they make conscious choices about which study behaviors to try, how much time to allocate to them, and when to modify their approach.

High performers accept that knowledge built gradually over time is fundamentally different from facts hastily memorized. They know that learning is an active process, and they devote the necessary time learning facts, struggling to understand how the facts relate to the big picture, creating knowledge, altering their mental models of what they know as they add new information, and they constantly strive to hone both their studying and test-taking skills. High performers devote a lot of time and effort through self-regulation to become so proficient.

This can be you because these are all skills that can be learned and practiced. Arguably, this section— *Practicing Your Skills*—is the most important in this book. We firmly believe that knowledge is power, especially when it relates to making substantial changes in some potentially deeply ingrained behaviors and habits. We want you to understand why we are telling you to do certain things; therefore, without going into a daunting level of detail, we first introduce you some fundamental concepts of memory (Chapter 7) and metacognition (Chapter 8) and then proceed to make some recommendations regarding study behaviors that tend to be the most effective (Chapter 9). Read these chapters slowly, and take a few notes. Reflect on the content by thinking about what it all means and how it applies to you. Be thinking about which of the methods you already use and how you might incorporate a few more into your repertoire.

Chapter 7

Learning to Perform

In 2000, Eric Kandel, a neuropsychiatrist, was awarded a Nobel Prize for his work on the cellular basis of learning. He demonstrated that during the learning process—the process of creating memories—individual neurons (nerve cells) alter both their structure *and* the way they are connected to other neurons (Medina, 2008; Sousa, 2006). It's utterly fascinating!

The way your brain adapts while you are learning is affected by numerous variables: the quantity of information and that rate at which it is presented to your brain, how you think about and process the information, as well as when and how often you review it. No wonder thinking is exhausting. The really great thing is that you, as a learner, have some control over how your brain is altered. Much like exercise improves your body, challenging your neurons in a deliberate manner improves your ability to study, think, learn, and remember.

Information comes to your brain through your five senses: you (1) see it, (2) hear it, (3) touch it, (4) smell it, or (5) taste it. Increased attention (mental focus) affords your brain the opportunity to more effectively and efficiently process this sensory information. In other words, when you pay attention, your ability to remember facts, understand concepts, and later use that information to solve problems is enhanced.

HOW DOES MEMORY WORK AND WHY DOES IT MATTER?

Your brain has a lot on its plate, so to speak. It is constantly bombarded by sensory information—the objects you are looking at, the sounds around you, the tactile sense of your clothing, the comfort of the chair you're sitting on, the itch on your left eyelid, the temperature of the room. Because there is so much information available to your brain, it has to make some decisions. What should it pay attention to? What can it ignore? What does it need to use right now? What does it need to store so that you will be able to use it later?

Take a moment to process the vast amount of information you could potentially be aware of at any given moment. Spend the next 30 seconds closely monitoring your five senses. What do you see? Smell? Hear? Feel? Taste? Then, go into another room and do something different for about one minute—stretch, get a drink of water, sing a song, anything you want. Before returning to your original location, try to remember everything you saw, smelled, heard, felt, and tasted during those 30 seconds of monitoring. Once you've remembered everything you can, return to your original location. How did you do? Was it easy? Was it hard? Do you think that closely monitoring your five senses helped you remember?

The way your brain deals with this information overload is by being selective—it only "pays attention" to some of it; the rest is filtered out. Although somewhat simplified, you could say the information entering your brain is handled in one of three ways: (1) used immediately then *discarded* (i.e., short-term memory), (2) stored in a location where it can be accessed and *recalled* at a later time (i.e., long-term memory), or (3) stored but cannot be retrieved, essentially lost (i.e., *forgotten*).

You may be asking yourself why you need to know this stuff. You may be thinking, I really don't care how my brain works and how memories are created. We believe that such thinking is a significant reason why some students study poorly—they don't know how memory works or they believe learning about how memory works will not improve their test scores. We strongly disagree!

Let's start with an analogy: Think of memory as a filing system, and the information from the five senses as notes jotted on pieces of paper.

You might throw away some of these notes, and keep others. Perhaps at some later time, you wish to find a note because there was something valuable written on it, but where do you look? People have different ways they file potentially useful papers. Some people keep them in piles scattered around the room and when they need to find one, they must make a time-consuming search through the piles. Other people have filing cabinets with file folders, and those folders are organized in some fashion, perhaps in chronological order, perhaps alphabetical by subject, or some other organizational system. The question is, which person is most likely to successfully locate the specific note in question?

One of your goals while studying is to develop a memory filing system that allows you to quickly find the scraps of information you've saved. Some people's brains, just like some people, tend to file information in a rather haphazard manner, analogous to the piles of paper strewn around a room. Quite often our brains file things alphabetically—"I remember it began with the letter 'M'"—and this can be helpful in some circumstances but not others. If you are trying to retrieve someone's name from memory, you can mentally flip through all the names that begin with the letter "M" until you find a "match." Taking this analogy one step further, we tend to think of certain names as being either boy names or girl names—in other words, we assign names to a broader category. This *association* between a name and a gender makes it even easier to recall someone's name if you know the first letter *and* you know whether they are a man or a woman; it allows you to generate a smaller number of possible correct names. If the person is a man, then you don't have to give Mary, Martha, or Michelle a second thought. This analogy illustrates (hopefully) the point that how you create your filing system and how you categorize, organize, and *associate* that information *while you study* can significantly aid in your subsequent recall of that information. This is one hugely positive outcome of effective study methods.

If you don't understand and/or choose not to apply these principles, you are likely to use study techniques that don't optimize your expenditure of time and effort. If you are interested in learning how to spend fewer hours studying yet attain higher scores on your upcoming tests, keep reading. If not, skip the rest of this section—however, we predict that if you do skip ahead, your test scores will not reflect what you are capable of achieving.

> **Critical Comment:** Improving your memory is dependent on your ability to focus on the task and organize information in meaningful ways.

PAY ATTENTION!

Sensory information that draws your attention and reaches your conscious awareness first enters your short-term memory (STM). From there, a subset of that information is transferred to your long-term memory (LTM). Some is discarded. Finally, and very importantly, at some later time, such as test day, you may need to retrieve the information from LTM in order to use it to answer a question, solve a problem, or make a decision (see Figure 7-1).

Before delving into a stimulating discussion of memory, we need to reiterate a very important concept—only the information on which you focus your attention enters your short-term memory *accurately*. Because individuals attend to different portions of all the available sensory information and may also organize it in different ways, two people can be present at the same lecture or read the same chapter in a textbook and have very different recollections based on which chunks of information were processed and transferred into their LTM. This is one reason why eyewitness testimony is not particularly reliable.

When you actively listen to music while reading, or study in a noisy coffee shop, or if you're eagerly waiting to receive a phone call or a text message—how much attention are you really directing toward what you are studying? If the sensory input is voluminous, it cannot all enter your STM memory for processing. In addition, the information

Figure 7-1

An Overview of How Memory Works

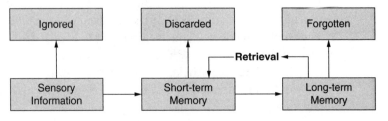

that does enter may not be of the highest quality and may or may not be relevant.

Multitasking diverts your attention through a process known as switch tasking. These repeated shifts in focus from one task to another result in information fragmentation, which produces processing inaccuracies and retrieval errors (Medina, 2008). Additionally, the process of switching between tasks takes much more time because your brain has to refocus after every switch. Your efficiency and effectiveness both suffer. Higher-scoring students study in distraction-free environments. Is this surprising? We hope not. The perils of multitasking were previously discussed in the chapter on time management (in Chapter 6); this chapter provides further explanation of the neurological reason why it's such a bad idea to multitask while studying. The next several pages describe in more detail the process of forming memories and provide suggestions on techniques you can use to develop a better memory.

STM

STM has two components—sensory memory and working memory (Mayer, 2010). Sensory memory preserves very briefly—in a few seconds or less—a highly-accurate representation of sensory information before some of that information is transferred to working memory (WM). WM converts these sensory "snapshots" into larger chunks of more organized information. For example, when someone tells you their phone number, very briefly the spoken sounds received via your ears are held in sensory memory until they enter your WM as recognizable numbers. This conversion makes the volume of sensory information easier to process.

STM has a very *limited capacity*, estimated to be about seven pieces of information. This limited capacity combined with the continuous stream of large volumes of information presented to your brain means your WM must process the chunks quickly and move them on. Information in WM has a *limited duration* of existence—estimated to be less than 30 seconds. In order to hold information in WM for a longer period of time you must rehearse it. This is why, when someone gives you a string of information such as a phone number, you either have to write it down, use it quickly, or repeat it to yourself over and over.

Ideally, as you study, all the relevant information from your WM would simply be transferred to your LTM. Unfortunately, this is not the case. In fact, a large amount of information simply passes through WM and is discarded, rather than stored.

If you're tempted to trivialize the role of STM in favor of LTM—after all, don't we want to remember things for more than 30 seconds?—by thinking of it as a mere temporary storage area or waiting room, don't. Although filing things in LTM is the ultimate goal of learning new information, STM is vitally important to our everyday functioning, reading accuracy, and problem-solving ability.

When faced with any situation or "problem" requiring a cognitive response, we must pull information out of our LTM back into our WM. Only once it's back in our WM can we manipulate the information and combine it with new data to solve a problem. Because WM has such a limited capacity, information pulled from LTM must compete for space with new data. Most people have pretty good long-term memories, once the information is "filed"; however, inadequate or underdeveloped STM can make learning very difficult. The good news is that through practice, you can improve both your working memory capacity and your processing capability. If you are thinking about what you are reading (and we know you are) your next question might be, how can I improve my memory?

Your memory is influenced by the quality (accuracy and relevance) of the information that enters your STM. To illustrate our point, here is a concrete example: Think of the first time you touched a hot stove (or perhaps you were spared this experience by a watchful mom. If so, just use your imagination). The sensory experience of touching the hot stove got your attention—the information reached your short-term memory accurately. It probably didn't take more than the one time to associate the hot stove with the sensation of pain. The unpleasant nature of the experience had meaning and relevance in your life, and the result was that in a single event you created a stable long-term memory. Not only that, you became capable of transferring that knowledge to different contexts, to different stoves in different kitchens. This is a classic example of how focus, understanding, and meaning combine to create a powerful memory. If only studying was that simple. Although it's not, it can come reasonably close if you use the right study techniques.

> **Critical Comment:** Emotions help you form memories. We are biologically programmed to form memories associated with emotional events, which is one reason why amusing anecdotes told by lecturers often stick with us. The flip side of this, however, is that a powerful emotional experience following a study session might actually interfere with the process of memory consolidation. So, for those of you who tend to unwind after studying by playing emotionally intense video games or engaging in some other emotionally stimulating activity, you might be undoing a great deal of hard work (Dworak et al., 2007).

LTM

As you study, sensory information enters your brain in the form of words, pictures, and sounds. To make this information available to you at a later time, your brain must attend to it, process it, and then transfer it from STM to LTM, where it is stored, more or less permanently. The process of converting sensory stimuli into LTM is called *consolidation*.

Information in your brain actually exists as electrical impulses transferred from one neuron (nerve cell) to another. Formation of a LTM is accomplished via (1) an acquisition process called encoding, and (2) a storage process called retention. A single memory involves physical connections called synapses and communication via electrical impulses between many neurons. Contrary to what might seem intuitive, a "memory" is not filed away as a unitary structure but is instead broken down into different components and the pieces stored in different places throughout the brain. The interconnected network of neurons activated together during memory consolidation is called a memory trace or engram. This memory trace is also activated when the memory is retrieved. Connectivity between neurons and groups of neurons is important for retention and retrieval.

The process of pulling information out of your long-term memory is known as retrieval. Once a long-term memory has formed, there is little, short of brain damage, that can eliminate it. Going back to our filing system analogy, once you've filed away a note by placing it in a pile or tucking it into folder and putting it into a filing cabinet, it's safely stored away, unless a fire destroys the room. More on forgetting in a moment.

Recognition versus Recall

Simply put, there are two types of retrieval: recognition and recall. Generally speaking, it is easier to recognize information than it is to recall it. Not all study methods improve recall; in fact, many common methods focus primarily on improving recognition. The problem is that not all exams are created equal in terms of whether they require recognition or recall to arrive at the correct answer. Figure 7-2 demonstrates how your memory helps you select the answer to a test question.

Some exams, such as essay and short answer, test your ability to recall information; others, such as multiple-choice exams composed of lower-order type questions merely require recognition. For example, suppose you are asked the following question: In what year did the Civil War begin? If you are provided no additional information, to answer the question you must recall the year from memory. Depending on how you first encountered, processed, and stored the information, you may or may not be able to retrieve the date from your memory when prompted in this manner. Those most likely to recall such a specific date probably have a strong connection to the information. Perhaps they're Civil War or history buffs, or maybe they learned the information fairly recently, or perhaps, when they studied it, they used a study method that helped them create a strong memory trace.

Figure 7-2

How Your Memory Works During the Test

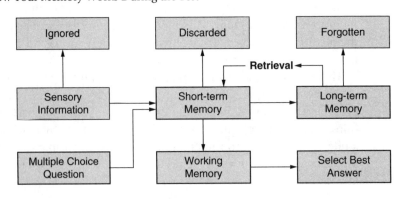

What if we take the same question, but turn it into a multiple-choice question with the following options: (1) 1561, (2) 1661, (3) 1761, (4) 1861, (5) 1961? Many people would now be able to answer it. We can often recognize a specific fact or detail when cues are available to trigger the memory. In the context of this question, some likely cues or memory triggers might include associating the date of the Civil War with something else of significance, such as Abraham Lincoln's presidency, or the century during which a majority of the states were forming, or that the Civil War began some time during the 1800s. Incidentally, it is probably already obvious to you that a question of this type would be made significantly more difficult by making the options more similar to each other: (1)1859, (2) 1860, (3) 1861, (4) 1862, (5) 1863.

STUDY TO IMPROVE RECALL

We want you to clearly understand the fundamental neurological difference between recognition and recall. Recognition is best thought of as a stimulus–response situation. The stimulus (a word or phrase in the test question) prompts your brain to make an association, which you then simply match to one of the options. Studying via repetition makes this process relatively easy. You practice the same thing over and over again. You rehearse it. You memorize the facts so well that when presented with the stimulus, the answer enters your working memory quickly. You may not understand it, but you do recognize it.

To use another analogy, picture what happens to a lawn when you walk on it, that is, the blades of grass are bent over by the weight of your feet. If you step on these blades of grass once, some might break, but others will merely bend and bounce back. If you then looked to find your footprints, there would be very little visible sign, and what little there was would disappear quickly. Now imagine that you walk that same path over and over, perhaps every day, as when you walk from your front door to the mailbox. After a while, you will see a visible path in the grass, perhaps you will have worn the grass down so much that you can see dirt. Forming memory traces is sort of like walking this path—the more times you revisit a memory, the easier it is to find your way back to it.

Recognition is an easier and quicker way to access information; unfortunately, it is a less helpful retrieval method for answering questions on standardized tests. The consequence of studying only for recognition is that you form relatively weak memory traces and very few neuron-to-neuron interconnections. You are prepared to answer questions that closely resemble how the information was originally presented to you—as we've said, fundamentally a matching process—but you are probably not able to use the information to solve novel problems or apply it in a different context. As discussed earlier in this book (hopefully you remember it), standardized tests are written to test you at higher cognitive levels (like those just mentioned) and generally provide fewer cues to help your recognize the correct answer. Most test-takers do well on teacher-generated tests because teachers typically provide multiple cues—both while teaching and on their tests. Because you will not have these cues for most standardized tests, you need to begin to train yourself for recall.

Recall is best thought of as a situation in which your ability to retrieve information is dependent not on a matching process but on the extent and strength of the memory trace. Imagine a memory trace that is represented by a larger, more interconnected network of neurons. This connectedness is the result of specific types of practice, for example, study methods. You need to expand your understanding of the concept of practice and not simply repeat the same thing over and over again. You need to approach the information from multiple perspectives. When you study for recall you prepare yourself to locate information filed away in your memory using any number of approaches—think of it as having many possible routes to the same destination—and all roads lead back to the memory. Chapter 9 describes more ways to help you do this well.

The result of studying for recall is that you are more likely to be able to recognize facts and concepts even when they are presented to you in a context different from how you originally encountered them; you remember the information for a longer time; you can apply the information to solve novel problems; and you can associate new information to what you already know, allowing you to learn and remember even more. To repeat ourselves yet again, standardized tests tend to assess your ability to answer higher cognitive level multiple-choice questions. Studying for recall increases the probability that you will be ready to do exactly that.

High-achieving students tend to use study techniques, such as elaboration and association, which allow them to attach powerful meaning to the information they learn, creating bigger, more interconnected neural networks and enhancing recall. *Elaboration,* as the name implies, involves adding details to help with understanding. Try to think of an example of something you've learned in which you realized you understood it better because it related to something in your personal life. Elaborating on information by thinking of its significance and meaning, its real-world application, and how it relates to things you already know, is a powerful learning method (Tigner, 1999).

Forming a*ssociations* creates meaningful links between newly acquired information and existing knowledge. Your ability to acquire, store, and use new information is improved by your ability to gather accurate sensory information and process it in your short-term memory, then *associate* it to previously stored information in your long-term memory. This is largely how adults learn, and it is why it is easier to learn very detailed information by building it up in layers over a period of time (as opposed to trying to cram all the details into a single study session).

Memory decay, the process of forgetting, is mostly about losing the ability to retrieve the memory—it's still there, you just can't find it anymore. Returning to the lawn analogy from before, imagine that you stopped walking to the mailbox day after day. Eventually, the grass would grow back and you wouldn't be able to see your footpath. The mailbox would still be there, but you might not be able to find it (well, you'd probably still be able to see it, but you get the picture, we hope). Think of the expression, "use it or lose it." Interestingly, the process of retrieval can strengthen a memory trace. This is actually one of the benefits of testing. Not only does testing "measure" how much you've learned, it also enhances your memory (Karpicke, Butler, & Roediger, 2009). You can use this principle while studying by frequently performing "free recall" exercises.

At this point, we hope we've conveyed the importance of the following ideas:

- Memory consolidation—transferring memory from short-term to long-term memory—is a primary goal while studying.
- Being able to retrieve stored information—pulling it out of LTM and into your working memory is key.
- You should be studying for recall, not simply recognition, so that you can use the information to answer higher-order questions.

REVISITING STUDY RESOURCES WITH MEMORY IN MIND

In Chapter 5—*Your Resources*—we distinguished between study aids and study behaviors. We defined *study aids* as materials you use to obtain content and *study behaviors* as the activities you engage in to build knowledge. The first two study behaviors—(1) thinking about the same thing in the same way and (2) thinking about the same thing in different ways—pertain specifically to study methods or techniques that help you acquire, transform, and process information. The balance of this chapter will introduce and explain some basic concepts about the use of study aids. In Chapter 8—*From Tactics to Strategy*—and Chapter 9—*Performance Enhancers*—we will expand on how you can develop different study behaviors and customize your study aids to make them uniquely helpful to you.

The good news is that many study aids and study methods can help you improve your memory and recall of information. Most people are familiar with the use of memory aids, known as mnemonics or mnemonic devices. These are typically single words or short phrases intended to aid in the recall of complex or voluminous information. A classic example from anatomy is the pseudo-chemical formula $LR_6SO_4 AR_3$. This mnemonic device is intended to help a student remember that the lateral rectus (LR) muscle of the eye is innervated by cranial nerve VI (6), the superior oblique (SO) muscle is innervated by cranial nerve IV (4), and "All the Rest" are innervated by cranial nerve III (3).

An acronym is another common type of mnemonic. This is generally a single word formed from the first letter of each item of a list. The acronym is easier to recall than the entire list. Because each letter of the word is associated with a specific item on the list, it acts as a powerful memory cue. A classic example is HOMES. This helps you remember the names of the Great Lakes: Huron, Ontario, Michigan, Erie, and Superior. You might also remember that we used the word "TEAMS" to stand for Time, Effort, Attitude, Motivation, and Selection.

Another classic example of a mnemonic device is the formation of a sentence. If you've taken music lessons, you might have used the mnemonic, "every good boy deserves favor" to remember the notes of the musical scale, E-G-B-D-F. The sillier (or funnier) the mnemonic, the better it functions as a memory device. However, be warned, simply trying to learn large quantities of information through the use of these devices is somewhat counterproductive. Memorizing a large number of mnemonics simply adds to the total amount of information you need to keep straight. We have worked with many students who used so many mnemonics they forgot what they stood for—they needed a mnemonic for their mnemonics.

Generally speaking, when trying to learn (remember) a large amount of complex information for the purpose of understanding and applying it, the creation and use of mnemonics should be considered a study method of last resort and be reserved for memorizing lists of details or the steps of a process, or some other similar task. To better assist you with improving your memory and increasing the effectiveness of your studying, the following section presents some ideas about study methods and study aids that will be of assistance in your quest to remember.

Avoiding the Illusion of Competence

We begin this section with a cautionary note—using study aids prepared by someone else is a study method that is too passive, which is not in your best interest. You need to get your hands dirty, so to speak. Study aids made by someone else might not emphasize important concepts *you* need to know, and they do not provide the opportunity for *your* brain to make the associations you need to make to aid your recall of the information. Even the best study aids made by someone other than you will not help you learn as much as something made by you. These other-created study aids helped the creator learn the information, but at best they will merely serve as a convenient package for you to memorize in a rote fashion. The key to effective study aids truly does lie in the "creative" aspect of making them. We will revisit this in the next two chapters, but you really need to understand the importance of this idea, so we repeat it once more with feeling: Study aids created by someone else *do not help you make the associations you need* to make in order for *you* to recall and apply the information.

Another pitfall of other-created study aids is that they tend to encourage skimming in a superficial manner and provide a sense of familiarity with the material, which is easily mistaken for knowing. As you review the study aid, you read words you have seen before, and you go through the material rather quickly because it is so familiar. You don't slow down to reflect on the information; you don't associate it with things you already know. On subsequent passes, you move through it even more quickly so you can cover more ground and feel good about how much you're accomplishing. Ultimately, you come to believe you know the material better than you actually do. Karpicke et al. (2009) refer to this as an "illusion of competence"; you mistake the fast pace at which you are able to progress through the information as knowledge. We see a great deal of this with the advent of recorded course lectures. Students tend to listen to these recordings on double speed, and they think that just because they can hear and understand most of the words being spoken they are also absorbing and processing the information.

Using Study Aids Effectively

Your use of study aids should be guided by two principles:

1. Use them with the *intent* of improving the effectiveness, not just the efficiency, of your studying.
2. Use them with the *intent* of creating stronger memory traces that will aid in your future recall.

We wish to draw your attention to the word "intent" in the foregoing principles. To be most beneficial, the selection, creation, and use of study aids must be purposeful, task specific, and driven by your learning goals.

A worthwhile step toward effective study is to transition from quantitative to qualitative learning goals, a topic that actually relates more to the next chapter—*Thinking About Thinking*. Goals provide a standard against which to measure your progress. Goals give you direction and provide motivation—they are an important key to accomplishment. Most students set study goals that focus on an "amount" of information to be covered, often measured in pages, "I have X number of pages to read by tomorrow." Although this is useful from a time management perspective, it cannot be the only way you measure your progress.

If you successfully achieve a quantitative goal—"Hooray, I read X number of pages!"—what is your measure of whether or not you actually learned anything? At some point it must cease to be about how many words pass over your eyes or into your ears; it's not even about how much you can actually stuff into your head, although making it into your head is a necessary first step. It's about the *quality* of the information that makes it in, and most importantly, it's about how much you can later retrieve and apply when answering test questions. Your selection of study aids and your decision about whether you choose other-created or self-created study aids should be guided by qualitative learning goals—what is the best tool to help you achieve the goal you've set for yourself?

Study aids can help you learn by:

- Focusing your attention on key concepts
- Condensing large volumes of complex information into smaller bundles of better organized, more simplified information
- Drawing attention to the associations between concepts
- Providing insight and meaning
- Developing your confidence in your ability to master the material

Study aids range from simple lists to complex diagrams. There are aids that help with rehearsal of information, aids for organizing information, and aids for crystallizing and clarifying patterns and complex interconnections among concepts. The simplest study aids represent abbreviated versions of complicated or voluminous information; examples include summary notes, outlines, and flashcards. These things facilitate rehearsal—reviewing something multiple times in exactly the same way. As we mentioned before, this allows you to reproduce the material exactly the way you memorized it for a short period of time. In much the same way as actors learn their lines, rehearsal methods allow you to replicate what you have memorized. And just as actors know what their next line is based on receiving the proper cue, such as the line of a coactor, you can provide the proper response on an exam question if and only if it provides you with the proper cue. What if you aren't given the familiar cue? Then suddenly you're like an actor forced to improvise. As most actors will no doubt tell you, improvising is not easy, and your ability to improvise is based on how well you understand the context of the situation. Generally, standardized tests are more similar to improvisation than a scripted production. Let's now turn our attention to a few of the more complex types of study aids.

- Outlines are a standard format used to organize and give structure to information in a way that highlights the hierarchical nature of relationships; their typical brevity can often depict at a glance the component parts as well as the whole. Three distinct limitations of outlines are that (1) they often lack sufficient detail, (2) they depict relationships as very linear or sequential when, in fact, the relationships might be better depicted as a web of interconnected facts and ideas, and (3) they can make it difficult to compare and contrast concepts located at different points in the outline.

- Charts, such as grids or tables, can be especially helpful in comparing and contrasting two or more concepts. Compare/contrast type questions are quite common on standardized tests. Selecting among options sometimes comes down to picking out "which one of these is not like the other ones."
- Flowcharts and decision trees allow you to see the steps involved in a procedure or process beginning from a specific starting point and navigating to the end of a series.
- Drawings and diagrams allow you to visualize complex relationships between facts and concepts, not readily accomplished in a more traditional outline.
- Finally, concept maps provide a more sophisticated way to visualize and understand complexity. A concept map combines elements of diagrams, tables, and flowcharts, and makes the associations among various ideas even more apparent. Concept maps are discussed further in Chapter 9.

Each of the study aids just described helps you organize and see the relationships between facts and concepts in different ways. By using memory-enhancing techniques such as elaboration and association, these progressively more complex and sophisticated study aids can help you remember and learn much more than mnemonics and simple rehearsal techniques. By creating these study aids yourself, you transform the information and make it your own, laying the foundation for building usable, flexible knowledge based on understanding, not memorization.

SUMMARY

In this chapter—*Learning to Perform*—we began with an overview of how memories are formed in order to better help you understand the important relationships between how you study, what you remember, and how you can use your memory to answer test questions.

Information enters our brain through our senses and this sensory information then proceeds to our STM. From there, and depending on what we pay attention to, some of this information makes it from our working memory (a component of STM) into our LTM. Once in LTM, forgetting is really a failure of the retrieval process—pulling information back out of LTM.

In Chapter 5, we commented that higher-scoring students tend to choose from among a greater variety of study resources, which they selectively use depending on the learning task before them. These students know that one study method or one study aid is not applicable in all situations. In our experience, higher-scoring students create their own study aids more often than other students. Additionally, their study aids tend to be more complete and robust.

We discussed the fact that study aids and study methods are not all equal in terms of how they prepare us to retrieve and apply information, and we provided reasons why studying for recognition is not enough. Studying for recall requires you to transform information to make it more meaningful to you, as well as more organized. Too often, "studying" becomes a passive process of highlighting and copying—such as copying notes—and repetitive rehearsal techniques such as flipping through flashcards or reading and rereading the same things over and over.

Transformation requires thought and action, such as annotating what you read, expressing ideas in your own words, manipulating information and elaborating on it to give it meaning, and associating new information to what you already know—does it confirm or challenge your prior knowledge—in order to truly "see" the interconnectedness of concepts and the relationships between details and principles.

Begin now to think about how you can transition away from just reading and reviewing toward reading, transforming, and thinking! Chapter 8—*From Tactics to Strategy*—will take you further down this path by showing you the value in learning to think about what you are thinking so that you can better change the way you think.

Before proceeding to Chapter 8, please reflect on the following questions:

- What was the primary take-away message for you from this chapter?
- What information will be the easiest for you to include in your exam preparation?

Be sure to complete the Chapter 7 Activity before starting to read Chapter 8.

CHAPTER 7 ACTIVITY

Improving your Ability to Remember

Chapter 7—*Learning to Perform*—presented an overview of how memory works and things that you can do to improve LTM and recall. Respond to the following prompts to gain a deeper understanding of how you can enhance your memory.

Table	
7–1	**Activity 1**

a. What can you do to create more meaning in what you are studying?

b. Compare and contrast recognition and recall.

c. Why will studying to improve recall improve your standardized test scores?

d. What can you do to reduce the possibility of developing an "illusion of competence"?

e. Provide two examples of association and elaboration using cars and bicycles.

8 From Tactics to Strategy

In Chapter 5 we introduced four categories of study behaviors: (1) thinking about the same thing in the same way, (2) thinking about the same thing in different ways, (3) managing your thinking, and (4) thinking about your thinking. We told you that *thinking about your thinking* is related to self-regulation and is a mental activity referred to as *metacognition*. Metacognition is generally described as self-knowledge regarding which learning strategies are most effective for a particular learning task or a problem to be solved.

SELF-REGULATION THROUGH METACOGNITION

Self-regulated learning includes making plans (selecting strategies, developing timelines) to achieve your learning goals, monitoring your progress, and modifying your behavior to keep you on track. Self-regulation requires metacognition (Brockkamp & Van Hout-Wolters, 2007; Ley & Young, 2001).

Before embarking on a mission to improve yourself, you need to establish goals, but before you can establish realistic goals, you must have an accurate assessment of your current capabilities. It would also be useful to have insight into what you would like to be able to do. The difference between your current level of ability and what you'd like to be capable of in the future defines your *performance gap*. For many, the most difficult part of setting achievable goals is identifying the magnitude of their performance gap. Failure to achieve this level of awareness is most often due to an inaccurate assessment of current ability. Many people are simply not very self-aware.

The Above-Average Effect

Most people have a propensity to overestimate their own ability. Not only are people overly *confident* in their self-assessment, they are absolutely certain they are more capable than reality suggests. Repeatedly, research shows that the average person rates themselves above average as compared to their peers—a statistical impossibility that has been called the "above-average effect." The tendency for very low performers to steadfastly believe they are more capable than they really are, in spite of abundant evidence to the contrary, is sometimes called the Dunning–Kruger effect, after the two researchers who published a landmark paper on the subject entitled, "Unskilled and unaware of it: how difficulties in recognizing one's own incompetence lead to inflated self-assessments" (Kruger & Dunning, 1999). Their argument, supported by research, is that incompetent individuals lack metacognitive or self-monitoring skills that would allow them to become aware of their own incompetence.

Before you can self-regulate you need to be able to accurately self-assess. Not surprisingly, based on our foregoing discussion, individuals who consistently tend to score the lowest on exams are commonly the least capable of assessing their own abilities (Kruger & Dunning, 1999; Regehr & Eva, 2006). *That does not mean they are bad people.* It means they are lacking an important skill set. Do you know anyone that might be lacking this important skill set? Is there any chance that you may lack this skill set? We wrote this book to help individuals preparing for tests to avoid this potential self-perpetuating trap.

Sometimes people who consistently overestimate themselves possess other very positive traits such as determination and perseverance—they don't give up easily. Unfortunately, because they are incapable of identifying their weaknesses, they tend to just keep trying. They either do more of the same thing, or they adopt a shotgun approach and try everything they can think of, to no avail. They have no strategy; all they have are ineffective tactics.

"Strategy" is a term borrowed from the military and is best thought of as a comprehensive plan developed with an eye toward accomplishing a specific goal. It includes within it a plan for obtaining feedback, monitoring progress, and making any necessary modifications to the overall plan. When an individual performs these steps in pursuit of their life goals, it is referred to as self-regulation. In the context of studying, you might define a tactic, in contrast to a strategy, as the use of a specific study aid. Low-performing students focus on tactics, whereas high-performing, self-regulating learners use strategy to achieve success, which is why we titled this chapter *From Tactics to Strategy*.

The Non-Self-Regulated Learner

Student A—we'll call him Pinot—is not a self-regulated learner. Pinot had to take the Graduate Record Examination to apply for graduate school. He had an undergraduate grade-point average (GPA) of 2.76/4.0 in engineering and wished to pursue a doctorate in electrical engineering at a prestigious university. To begin his preparation, he asked Suzy, a philosophy major, what she did to prepare for the exam because he knew she scored in the 90th percentile in all areas. Even though Suzy had a different undergraduate major, a better GPA, as well as a different educational background, different life experiences, different interests, and a very different personality, Pinot bought the same review books Suzy had used and studied for the same number of weeks that Suzy did, but achieved a very low score—below the 5th percentile. Pinot was surprised at his score and surprised at how hard the analytical thinking and vocabulary sections of the exam were. What did Pinot do wrong?

The Self-Regulated Learner

Student B—we'll call this student Syrah—is a self-regulated learner. Syrah had a 3.8/4.0 GPA in human biology and had to take the Medical College Admission Test (MCAT) to apply to a well-respected medical school. Syrah began her preparation process by logging onto the MCAT website to more learn about the exam. She also talked to the premed advisor at her university to find out if he could offer any helpful hints regarding test-taking skills—the thought of taking such an important standardized test was causing her some anxiety. He referred Syrah to the counseling center, so Syrah made an appointment and learned some anxiety reduction techniques. Syrah then thought about which subject areas she had the most difficulty in and realized that her worst grades were in English. She felt she didn't have a very strong vocabulary and knew her reading skills needed work. Syrah asked several other human biology majors, who had been accepted into medical school, what they had done to prepare. She then went to the bookstore to look at the books they'd recommended to see which ones seemed to cover the material in a way that would help her the most. She ended up buying four different review books, none of which had been recommended by the people she had talked to. Syrah knew that she learns best when information is presented with many examples and practice questions, but she also knew that she had to improve her reading speed and comprehension, so she skipped over the review books that contained mostly outline-formatted information and purchased more comprehensive review books in biology, chemistry, and physics, as well as a vocabulary question book. Syrah then created a study plan to cover the time period until her exam and divided her time between doing practice questions and refining her weak areas. Syrah did very well, scoring at or slightly above the 85th percentile in each of the three main areas covered on the exam. What did Syrah do right?

LEARN TO GET AND USE FEEDBACK

The best way to arrive at an accurate assessment of your current ability is to obtain feedback from as many sources as possible. You can't just sit back, think about how smart you are, and decide you're better than most. You need to use multiple "assessment tools" to get as complete a picture as possible. What's your GPA? What's your class rank? How do you generally perform on examinations—barely pass, middle of the range, highest score in the class? These things provide more objective data. Like it or not, performance data are correlated with academic success. What type of feedback or evaluations do you get from people you've interacted with? Positive? Negative? Mixed bag? Don't limit your feedback to that from close friends, relatives, or people who only say "nice things." You can't *just* ask your mom and best friend (although you should ask them too). Solicit the opinion of teachers, advisors, coaches, mentors, bosses, coworkers, teammates, siblings, parents, friends, and other people who know you well. All this feedback is subjective, but if you obtain enough of it, the complete picture will be more accurate. Make sure you explain why you are asking and request that they provide honest, candid feedback. Then, and very importantly, *listen* to what they tell you and *think* about it. Thank them for their time and opinion, and avoid becoming defensive. Don't respond by making excuses or telling them why you believe their observations are wrong. Remember, this is for your own good.

The more feedback you acquire, the more you pay attention to and reflect on what you hear, the more you compare the judgments and evaluations of others to how you perceive yourself, the more likely you'll draw an accurate picture of your current abilities—strengths and weaknesses. When you think about and evaluate how you think, you become better at thinking. By obtaining feedback from a variety of sources you can begin to make improvements based on data, not hopeful thinking (Bice & Sefcik, 2010).

Applying Metacognition in Exam Preparation

Metacognition involves understanding and awareness of your own mental and cognitive processes, hence "thinking about thinking" or "knowing about knowing." Although it seems like a very esoteric concept, it includes eminently practical activities such as using awareness of your strengths and weaknesses to plan an approach to a task. Most people use metacognitive processes every day. Even something as simple as knowing whether or not you know how to get to where you're going requires metacognition; for example, if you have to drive to someone's house for a party. Someone who denies that they're lost, even when it's patently obvious they don't have a clue where they are, is not using metacognition.

It is through metacognition that you come to appreciate what you already know and what you still need to learn in order to accomplish a particular task or achieve a specific goal. Effective metacognition helps you make good decisions through accurate and purposeful monitoring of your current state of knowledge. It is through meta-cognitive processes that you determine which learning activities will increase your proficiency. Thinking about your own thought processes enables you to gain the self-awareness necessary for effective self-regulatory behaviors: planning, monitoring, and adapting.

Hopefully, we've made our point: metacognition is extremely important during exam preparation. Essentially metacognitive processes function like someone in your head (you) constantly asking you questions:

- "Am I learning this material?"
- "Do I know this?"
- "How do I know this?"
- "Am I 100% certain?" "90%?" "50?" "Just guessing?"
- "Am I on the correct path toward success?"
- "What is the most important content for this examination?"
- "Do I need to adopt different study methods for my exam preparation?"
- "Do I need to adjust the pace of my preparation?"

And so on. With monitoring and reflection also comes evaluation of your learning process and some additional questions:

- "So far, has my plan of preparation been more or less effective than I had expected?"
- "What can I do differently?"
- "What do I need to review again to fill in blanks or gaps in my preparation?"

Taking time to develop metacognitive knowledge, rather than always focusing on specific examination content, sets the expert learner apart from the novice learner. When difficulties arise in preparation for an examination, the expert learner stops and reflects on their experience and analyzes what has been effective and what needs to be modified. If they recognize a problem, but don't know how to resolve it, they seek guidance from someone who is in the position to know, an author-ity, an expert. That last is an important point: *it's not that self-regulated learners always know the right thing to do, it's that they recognize when they don't and they do something about it.* Novice learners often lack this awareness and continue to use the same tactics over and over again. This results in repeated failures and triggers other impediments to successful examination preparation such as test anxiety, negative thoughts, or procrastination.

Develop Metacognitive Skills with the Monitor-Reflect-Evaluate-Modify Approach

Like any other skill, you can improve your metacognition through deliberate practice. One approach is the use of a process diary, a structured format used to record what you are doing and thinking. An advantage of recording this information is that it allows you to review your progress without relying on your memory, which might be faulty. Keeping a diary allows you to track your experiences, develop a way to measure what you are doing, reflect on your progress, think about and evaluate what you have been doing, and determine what you need to change (review and complete the Chapter 8 Activity). Using "self-talk" can supplement your process diary. Self-talk, or "thinking aloud," rather than keeping the thoughts inside your head, makes your metacognitive processes more obvious to you. By listening to yourself, you are more likely to notice errors, biases, exaggerations, or inconsistencies in your thinking.

Step #1, Monitor: To begin your self-improvement process you must actively monitor what you do and "measure" how well you do it. Before you can change, you have to know where you stand. If you don't monitor what you do, how can you identify what you need to improve? Furthermore, if you don't have an established baseline for comparison, how will you know if you have, in fact, improved?

Step #2, Reflection: After you collect some data the next step is to think about it. Reflection requires that you stop what you're doing in order to think about what you're doing.

Step #3, Evaluate: Reflection allows you the opportunity to evaluate your performance. What worked? What didn't?

Step #4, Modify: The final step in this metacognitive sequence is to modify your behavior, strategy, or tactics, if necessary. Once you know what you have been doing (by monitoring it) and how well you have been doing it (through reflection and evaluation), you're ready to change.

SUMMARY

High performers are typically self-regulated learners. They are goal-driven and they approach learning tasks with a strategy. Self-regulation requires a mental skill set, collectively referred to as metacognition. Simply defined, metacognition is "thinking about thinking" or "knowing about knowing." It is the ability to self-monitor and self-assess. Most people overestimate their abilities, and consistently low scorers on examinations are often the same ones who most steadfastly believe they are more capable than they really are.

Developing a more accurate self-assessment requires obtaining feedback from a number of different sources, some more objective and quantitative, such as GPA, class rank, and previous exam scores, and some more subjective and qualitative, such as the opinions of people who know you. It is important to evaluate this feedback and compare it to your own self-assessment. If your assessment differs from the picture generated from a wide variety of other sources, it is at least probable that your assessment is flawed.

To advance your ability to study, learn, and apply your knowledge most effectively, it is important you go beyond study behaviors that focus on content knowledge and develop higher cognitive skills, such as metacognition. We suggest keeping a process diary, perhaps combined with self-talk, and using the monitor-reflect-evaluate-modify process to help you move from tactics to strategy when preparing for your standardized exam.

Before proceeding to Chapter 9, please reflect on the following questions:

- What was the primary take-away message for you from this chapter?
- What information will be the easiest for you to include in your exam preparation?

Be sure to complete the Chapter 8 Activity before starting to read Chapter 9.

CHAPTER 8 ACTIVITY

Creating a Process Diary

In Chapter 8—*From Tactics to Strategy*—we introduced the concept of using a diary as an effective means of enhancing metacognition. Using the questions listed below as a guideline reflect upon your thinking. Note your awareness of your thought processes and comment on how you are dealing with each of the situations listed below. Each day, add any additional comments about your thoughts as you become more aware of how you think about your thinking. It is important to write as much as possible, as frequently as possible to enhance your metacognition knowledge.

Table	
8–1	**Activity 1**

a. How did my learning go today?

b. Do I have a clear understanding of what I am doing?

c. Were there thoughts that were distracters that slowed my learning?

d. How can I attack learning challenges more efficiently and effectively?

e. What tactics are working? How can I modify any tactics that are not working well?

f. Am I planning effectively? How are my thoughts helping or hindering?

Chapter

9 Performance Enhancers

We introduced Section III—*Practicing Your Skills*—by declaring it the most important section in this book. The two chapters you just read (7—*Practicing Your Skills*; 8—*From Tactics to Strategy*) and their associated activities serve as a springboard for this one—*Performance Enhancers*—arguably the most important chapter in Section III. To maximize your performance, you need to take your skills to the next level; performance enhancers will help you do just that. Achieving the highest score possible on your upcoming test will be determined, to a large extent, by how well you master the information presented in this chapter and apply it to your subsequent studying.

In our experience, individuals who score the highest on standardized tests share some common characteristics: They possess accurate insight and realize when their choice of study techniques is not allowing them to perform to their maximal potential (metacognition). They are motivated to study by the satisfaction they derive from learning (intrinsic interest). They are confident in their ability to succeed and believe that failure represents an opportunity to learn from their mistakes (high self-efficacy). They have a written study plan, they accurately monitor their progress, and they update it regularly (self-regulating). Finally, *they know how and when to employ a variety of different study techniques*. It is this last issue—the appropriate application of the best study techniques at the right time for the right task—that is the primary focus of this chapter.

Examinees that score the lowest on standardized tests are often very good at memorizing material and typically devote a significant number of hours studying for their tests; hence, they often know a lot of facts and information. If they know so much, then why do they not score higher? The answer lies in the questions they use to guide their studying—the "what–what" dyad. The first "what" is necessary; it represents content, as in, what do I need to study? The second "what" is misleading; it represents questions such as these: *What's the secret? What do I need to do to score higher? What can you tell me so that I can pass?* Individuals need to move past this second "what." It's far too passive; there is no good answer to be given for this "what" question. They need to take a more active role, get rid of the "what–what," and replace it with "why and when."

Higher-scoring examinees actively seek the "why and when"? The "why" includes *Why does this fact matter? Why should I know this? Why did all those hours I studied for my last test not pay off?* Higher-scoring examinees use "why" questions to provide direction and regulation to their future studying, and to challenge themselves to broaden the scope and depth of what they are learning.

The "when" includes the following: *When should I use this fact or information? When does "technique A" lead to outcome "B" and are there other times when "technique A" could lead to outcome "C" or "D"? When I use study technique "X" instead of technique "Y" will my score improve (if not, then why)?* Higher-scoring examines use "when" questions to help them associate and elaborate. You might recall that making associations and using the technique of elaboration help you build strong memory traces and better enable you to retrieve information from your memory. The more information that is interconnected in your memory—links between different pieces of information—the easier it is to recall information when confronted with a different or novel stimulus (i.e., memory cue); in essence, you have multiple pathways to the stored memory. High-scoring individuals use "when" questions to challenge themselves to expand the connectivity of what they are learning.

More than 50% of the questions on standardized tests will ask you to apply your knowledge in a manner or context fundamentally different from the one in which you studied it (Crooks, 1988; Gall 1984; Jandaghi & Shaterian, 2008; Larsen, 2006; Zheng, Lawhorn,

Lumley, & Freeman, 2008). The ability to use information learned in one context to answer a question framed in a novel context is an important skill known as *transfer* (Ambrose et al., 2010). Practice is required to develop the ability to transfer information from the context in which it was learned to a different context presented in a test question. You need to learn to think creatively and flexibly about what you are learning, and this is where performance enhancers come in.

"Getting the main idea"—do you remember that from elementary school? Our teachers instructed us that this was an important basic reading skill—to be able to read a passage and understand the gist of it. Guess what, they were right. Unfortunately, not everyone learned this skill, and some went entirely the other way. Some learned to get the main idea quite well, but never went beyond that point. Once you "get" the main idea or central theme of what you're reading, which represents the commonality that binds the information together—the point, the purpose, the big picture—then you need to understand how the facts and details fit together and support the main idea. Learning is not usually an either-or proposition. You need to practice both, and you cannot do that through rehearsal strategies alone.

The ability to interrelate facts, details, concepts, ideas, and principles requires multiple perspectives and the use of integrative studying and thinking techniques. Lower-level learning focuses on the facts, details, and particulars, while higher-level learning directs more attention to principles and concepts and the relationships among them and the supporting facts and details. You need to achieve this higher level of thinking.

To help you move from lower-level thinking to higher-level thinking, this chapter is divided into three areas: (1) reading skills, (2) self-testing techniques, and (3) group studying. These techniques build on each other and should be used in the sequence in which they are described for optimal results. The skills will help you learn to use specific study techniques to move purposefully from lower-level memorization to higher-level critical thinking and problem solving.

READING SKILLS

When some people read a book or an article, they tend to skim through it without actively reading it. It's a little like riding in a boat, gliding over the surface of the water; you're on the water, but you're not in the water. When you study, you need to swim; you need to become immersed. Some students tell us that to save time they have been taught to read only the first and last sentences of a paragraph because "the first sentence introduces the content of the paragraph and the last sentence summarizes it"—so why bother reading all the stuff in the middle, that's just detail, right? Why bother? Because the information that will help you associate the material, remember it, and ultimately help you apply it, is usually "all that stuff in the middle." The stuff in the middle is the meat on the bones, the substance, the specifics; it's what provides meaning, significance, and support for the main idea.

SQ4R

Robinson described the SQ3R (SQRRR) reading technique as a method to improve reading comprehension (Johns & McNamara, 1980; Robinson, 1970). It is a useful technique for individuals at every level of reading skill, especially when reading complex information. The five-letter acronym stands for *Survey, Question, Read, Recite,* and *Review*. When some students "read" they never even get to the first "R," but rather default to "S"—they survey or skim the material but don't ever really read it. In contrast, most high-achieving students tend to progress through all five steps and sometimes add a sixth step (letter); a fourth R signifies "Reflect" (Thomas & Robinson, 1982) or "Relate" (Simpson & Nist, 2000). Yes, it takes them longer to get through the material but that's what makes them high scorers. They are purposeful and deliberate in their approach. Read on to learn how you can do this too.

Survey

Each time you study new material, begin by Surveying (S) what you are going to read. Your goal is to obtain an overview, a lay of the land, so to speak. It's like walking into a room and glancing around to see what the room is used for, what's in it, who's in it, and what *you* might use it for. Take some time to flip through the chapter or article or handout, whatever it is. Read the headings and the boldfaced text, read the legends on the figures, graphs, tables, and charts. Don't try to memorize any of the information at this stage. Evaluate how it's formatted and presented. Does the presentation start with a more general perspective and move toward specific examples, or does it start with a specific example then proceed to general principles? Is the organization similar to an expanded outline with major headings, minor headings, and so on? Is it divided into sections? Get a sense of how much there is to read and estimate how long it will take you to thoroughly read it. Will you be able to realistically read it in one session or will you need to divide it into smaller chunks? Where are the good stopping points? It is only during this "S" stage—your initial encounter of the material—that you should skim. This should not take you very long.

Question

After you have completed your preliminary survey of the chapter, pause and ask yourself some questions. Here are some examples to get you started brainstorming:

- I wonder what I will learn? Try to guess.
- I wonder what the author is trying to convey? Speculate.
- How might I apply this material later? Use your imagination.
- What key elements should I focus so I can understand the rest? Be logical.
- How will this relate to what I already know or will read later? Associate.

The point of this stage is to frame what you are about to read and prepare your brain to be looking for answers. A brain learns best when it's given a goal—it treats the reading like an information treasure hunt—the suspense is riveting: will you or won't learn the answers to your questions? The more you practice this brainstorming technique, the better you will become at asking the kinds of questions that will greatly enhance the actual reading process.

Read, Recite, Review, and Relate

When you read the material, do it *slowly* and *thoroughly*. Read for detail; don't skim, don't omit, don't skip around. Keep distractions at bay and focus on the text. If the reading material is brief or not particularly dense (less than 30 minutes of reading time), read it all the way through. If it's longer than that, break it into 20- to 30-minute chunks.

Once you've read all or part of it, stop and try to recite or recall it from memory, take notes, try to summarize what you've just read to the best of your ability. The important part of this stage of the SQ4R process is that you do this from memory. This is a form of self-testing. The memory retrieval process will actually help to strengthen the memory traces that were formed, making it much easier to recall the information later. This will also help you to identify the gaps in your knowledge. Don't be surprised if you tend to better remember what you read first and last than the stuff in the middle—this is referred to as the primacy and recency effect, a cognitive bias that we will discuss again in Chapter 11. By pausing to recite, every half hour or less, you can prevent yourself from studying too long before realizing you haven't been paying attention. Reading for hours and hours without break has the potential to waste a lot of time if you have no recollection of what you've been reading. If you find yourself struggling to maintain focus, begin by reading for only 10–15 minutes before you pause to recite.

After your recitation, go back to the text and review. Compare your notes to the reading. What did you remember? What did you forget? As you review the text, supplement your notes with more details and embellish them using elaborative strategies and associations to create connections and integrate the new knowledge with the old—this is the fourth "R," relate. What does this information remind you of? How does it relate to the real world? How does it apply to you? What new words did you learn? How can you begin to use them in your everyday life?

This six-step approach (SQ4R) to reading can be daunting initially, and it will take longer to complete than a single, quick, one-time read, or skim-through. However, the dividends—better long-term memory, more complete recall, and ultimately the ability to transfer—are well worth the extra effort and time.

In preparation for learning about your next performance enhancer, pause, jot down some notes, review the last few pages, relate the last few pages to previous material in the book, take a break, and then continue reading.

From Words to Pictures

As we discussed in Chapter 5, creating study aids to organize new information and to associate it with your existing knowledge is a powerful study technique. A great way to do this is through the creation of visual aids—tree diagrams, flow charts, and concept maps—that connect facts, details, and concepts, clearly demonstrating their relationships. Creating these visual representations helps you engage in active learning processes; no longer are you just reading or reviewing, you are organizing and building.

Concept mapping (and a related, but different, process known as mind mapping) is a sophisticated method of building a two-dimensional image to display relationships between concepts and facts (West, Pomeroy, Park, Gerstenberger, & Sandoval, 2000). Concept maps can range from fairly simple to extremely complex. A concept map is basically a hierarchical or weblike visual representation of the structure of a body of knowledge. A very basic concept map begins with a central or core idea, possibly a question—what is a shape or why is grass green? This central idea is connected to major themes or concepts, each referred to as a domain of knowledge, by drawing lines between them. Each domain is further connected by lines to other, related components—other concepts, principles, and details (see Figure 9-1).

Figure 9-1

Basic Concept Map

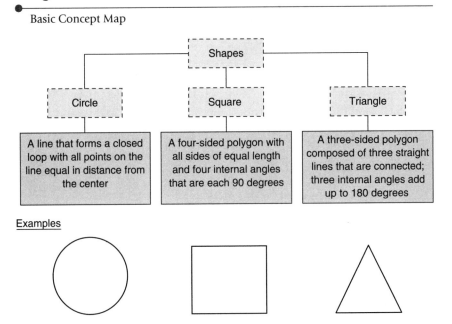

Examples

The more advanced your understanding of the knowledge domain, the more ways you will be able to draw a concept map of the same material and the more cross-linkages your maps will include. Cross-linkages represent associations and relationships among key concepts and visually connect information across domains; cross-links are sometimes represented by dashed lines. The more associations you make, the more complex and interconnected your map, moving from a simple branching tree diagram (Figure 9-1) to something more resembling a web (Figure 9-2). Ultimately, identifying and understanding these cross-linkages are the goals of concept mapping. This study method will assist you in understanding complexity and will help you build strong memory traces, enabling you to more effectively recall and transfer your knowledge.

SELF-TESTING TECHNIQUES

Most students study using rehearsal methods. Some students use rehearsal methods exclusively. Rehearsal can indeed help you memorize

Figure 9-2

Concept Map with Cross-Linkages

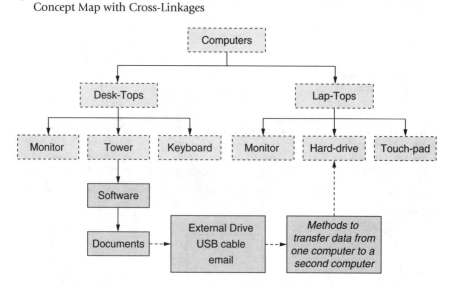

material, but that's not good enough. As discussed in Chapter 7, you should anticipate encountering content presented in different, perhaps unfamiliar, contexts. This will be true of over 50% of the questions on a standardized test. These exams test your ability to apply (*transfer*) what you know. Being able to recognize information isn't enough. Even being able to recall information isn't quite enough, although, it's one step closer. You need to be able to *apply* what you know.

Here is a very rudimentary example of what we mean by testing the application of knowledge, versus simply testing knowledge.

Sample Knowledge Question: What is the wavelength of green light?

A. 650 nm
B. 475 nm
C. 570 nm
D. 510 nm
E. 400 nm

This question simply requires you to have memorized that the wavelength of green light in 510 nm.

Sample Application Question: Green is to grass as blue is to _____.

A. Sky
B. Water
C. Ball
D. Sad
E. Moon

This question requires you to recognize the relationship of green to grass, understand the physics concept that color is due to the type of interaction (e.g., absorption or reflection) between different wavelengths of light in the visible spectrum and various materials, and know that grass is green because it reflects green light, just as a ball is blue because it reflects blue light. The sky and water are blue for different reasons pertaining to the physics of light, and the options "sad" and "moon" reflect a totally different type of relationship to color. In this case, memorizing the wavelengths of various colors does not help you answer the question.

Learning to use self-testing techniques is an excellent way to begin to apply your knowledge. We will present two basic methods of doing this: writing your own test questions and practicing using prepared question-and-answer (Q&A) resources.

WRITING YOUR OWN TEST QUESTIONS

Writing your own test questions is an excellent way to prepare (King, 1992). Not only can it help you learn to anticipate what you might be asked, but it's also an excellent way organize your thoughts and solidify your understanding of material. As you write your own questions, you'll compare and contrast facts and concepts, you'll learn to analyze information and develop an appreciation for nuance and complexity, and you will see very clearly the difference between testing knowledge of a fact versus testing application of a concept. All of this will greatly enhance your preparation.

Write questions as if you were a teacher planning to assess the understanding of your students. How would you be sure they knew the content? How would you assess whether they can apply what they know? Once you've constructed the question, what options will you provide? In addition to the correct answer, what would you include as your distractors? By writing your own questions you will increase your understanding and improve your memory. Win–win, yes?

As you write your "test," avoid creating low-level items (e.g., knowledge-based recall questions that simply test facts, definitions, etc.). This would be a waste of your time. Instead, do your best to write higher-order questions. Write questions that would challenge an examinee; questions that require analysis and evaluation of information. Write questions that require the examinee to apply what they know, not just demonstrate they can recognize facts.

To write good questions that will augment your studying we recommend you include three basic question components: (1) a stem, (2) an interrogatory, and (3) four or five answer options (see Figure 9-3). The stem presents information needed by the examinee to select an answer. It can be short, consisting of just a phrase or a sentence or two, or it can be a paragraph or more in length. It could include data in the form of a table, chart, drawing, or graph. The interrogatory poses the "question" to be answered and helps direct the examinee's thinking. The stem and the interrogatory both need to be written so the examinee can understand exactly what is being asked of them. If the question

Figure 9-3

Basic Structure of a Multiple-Choice Question

STEM	A college student enters a national forest at the southern entrance. After 45 minutes of hiking off-trail he realizes he has lost his way. The forest is filled with trees, creeks, animals, and unmarked trails and paths. The day is heavily overcast with intermittent rain showers.

INTERROGATORY	Which of the following is the best method for this student to use to orient himself in the forest?

ANSWER OPTIONS	A. Listen for the hoot of an owl. B. Find a creek and assess the direction of water flow. C. Identify where the moss is growing on any trees that have moss growing on them. D. Look for a path. E. Use his shadow to determine directionality.

is ambiguous or vague, it will be unnecessarily challenging. Learning to write good stems and interrogatories isn't easy, but the challenge will improve your learning of the material as well as your preparation to answer these types of questions on exam day. Granted, this study method does take time, and it's not likely you will use it if your current exam is scheduled for next week, but try it for next time.

Once you've written the stem and the interrogatory, you need to create the answer options. Each of the four or five options usually falls into one of two categories: (1) a correct answer (keyed answer) and wrong answers (distractors) or (2) the best answer (keyed answer) and partially correct answers (distractors). Because most standardized tests are created using higher-level questions, it is unlikely that you will be asked to identify the correct answer; standardized tests ask for the best answers (see Figure 9-4). Challenging examinees to identify the best answer assesses their ability to interpret data, verify their understanding of information, and weigh evidence to make decisions. When you write your own questions, keep this in mind. Design your questions to challenge the examinee to differentiate between the best answer to the question and other options that contain some correct information but are not the best answer. The better you can train yourself to recognize

Figure 9-4

Answer Options for Lower-Level and Higher-Level Questions

	Keyed Answer	Distractors
Lower-Level Questions	Right Answer	Wrong Answers
Higher-Level Questions	Best Answer	Partially Correct Answers

subtle differences in information, the less you will see challenging questions as "tricky questions."

There are very few absolutely incorrect options. That might not make much sense to you, so let us try to explain. Factual information is surrounded by the contextual elements of the question stem, and depending on your interpretation of the question and its context, you could potentially select an answer that is not appropriate for the context of the question. It might be a true or correct statement, but it doesn't answer the question being asked. It might be right some of the time, but not right in this instance. For example, the same object will weigh less on the moon than it does on earth. If you were given a question that required you to determine the weight of an object with a specific mass, and the question specified "on the moon," but you either overlooked that part, or didn't realize that it mattered, and the options included both the weight of the object on earth and the weight on the moon, you might select the weight on earth, even if you essentially performed the correct calculation. Context.

Which answer did you select in Figure 9-3? If you chose "C" because you knew that moss grows on the north side of trees, good for you! If you chose "C" because you didn't know the answer but recognized that it is the longest answer and knew that longest answers are recommended choices when guessing, good for you. If you chose another answer for a different reason, you should find Chapter 11—*Maximizing Your Points*—very helpful. In Chapter 11 we discuss some test-taking skills to help you select answers even when you have no clear idea what the best answer might be.

How can you begin to transition your study techniques toward this more involved and elaborate method? One suggestion is to take something you might normally do—take notes or create outlines or flashcards—and challenge yourself to covert note taking into question writing. Instead of highlighting a textbook, create a test item for those important details, ideas, or concepts.

PRACTICING USING PREPARED QUESTION-AND-ANSWER (Q&A) RESOURCES

Practice *doesn't* make perfect; only the right kind of practice makes perfect. Deliberate practice is what fosters improvement and expertise (Colvin, 2010; Ericsson, Prietula, & Cokely, 2007). This is true of all things in life. If you want to learn to ride a bike, you don't go waterskiing. If you want to improve your reading skills, you don't do math problems. If you want to improve your math skills, you don't study anatomy. Get the picture? To get good at something, you have to practice doing what it is you want to get good at. Furthermore, you want to plan your practice, make sure you're doing the right things based on your current skill level, and you need to obtain feedback on your progress.

If you're preparing for a standardized multiple-choice exam, then one of the things you need to do is practice answering multiple-choice questions. But not just any questions are optimal. If you're studying for the Medical College Admissions Test doing practice questions written for the Graduate Record Examination is not going to help you (or not help you as much). Additionally, there's some logic to matching the questions you do to your current learning goal. We will address this in our discussion of using questions to learn content, using questions to understand context, and using questions to obtain feedback. Using questions in these three different ways either in succession or in some iterative fashion, throughout your studying, will provide you maximal benefit.

How can you improve the utility of practice questions during your preparation process? First, let's take a look at the standard drill:

1. Read the question quickly.
2. Try to figure out the right answer as quickly as possible.
3. (a) Peek at the correct answer or (b) don't peek at the correct answer. Record your response.
4. Move on to the next question and repeat.
5. Do as many questions as is humanly possible.
6. Tally your score.

7. If you are feeling particularly motivated, hastily skim the explanations provided—why the right answer was right and the wrong answers were wrong.

In our experience, that's usually the sum total of how people view the function of practice questions—drill, drill, drill. Do you want to do better?

We maintain that there are many reasons for using prepared Q&A resources and many ways to use them. We will discuss four of these: (1) honing your question writing and question analysis skills, (2) learning content, (3) appreciating context, and (4) obtaining feedback (to improve the quality of your content knowledge, your problem-solving abilities, and your self-regulatory skills).

Honing Your Question-Writing and Question-Analysis Skills

As you use Q&A resources to study, imagine how you would modify the questions to make them different or even more challenging. How might you edit a stem so that it provided less information (hence, fewer memory cues) and forced the examinee to recall more from memory and draw more conclusions for themselves (i.e., make it a higher-level question)? How might you change the interrogatory to make one of the other answer options a better answer? How might you edit the options to make a wrong answer the right answer, a partially correct answer a better answer, the keyed answer a less correct answer? In this way, you challenge yourself to take a single question and create many other possible questions.

Learning Content

Learning content from Q&A resources is a very common exam preparation tactic. Some students even read Q&A books just as they would read a review book. They try to memorize the content, hoping that if they see the same or comparable question on the test, they will recognize it and "get it right."

If you are just beginning to study for this exam, this can be a fruitful way to learn some content, under certain circumstances. If the multiple-choice questions you are reviewing are very fact-based, you may in fact learn some new information using this method. However, if you already know a reasonable amount of content, reading or answering fact-based (i.e., low level) items, will not be of much value to you. On the other hand, if your current level of content knowledge is still fairly weak, then reviewing higher-level items can be very frustrating, discouraging, and confusing.

What do we recommend? If you are just starting to study, supplement your studying with lower-level fact-based multiple-choice questions. Once you gain a reasonable appreciation of the breadth of the content, then you need to start to use the multiple-choice questions to help you appreciate context.

Appreciating Context

After you have done some reading and produced stacks of annotated notes and pages of concept maps, it's time for you to start using multiple-choice questions to appreciate context. To do this well, you need a Q&A resource, such as a book or computer-based resource that provides higher-level multiple-choice questions. Most standardized exams, especially national exams, have specific Q&A resources designed specifically for practice. Some of these are hard-copy books, some are software-based, and some are Web-based. Web-based resources often require paying a subscription fee for a certain period of time. Any of these will do, but make sure you do a little research on your exam so that you can purchase the appropriate types of questions—you want them to be similar to the actual test items.

There are two ways to use multiple-choice questions to gain broader context. (1) Organized by specific content area or discipline (e.g., biology, math, physics, anatomy, physiology, chemistry, or history). Make sure you consult a test blueprint for your specific exam. (2) Organized randomly in the form of a comprehensive practice test. The advantage of working through multiple-choice questions organized by discipline, or a specific topic within a discipline, is that it helps you focus on one subject at a time, which might help you broaden your knowledge of the topic. A rather substantial disadvantage is that these types of questions are often very similar to one another and they don't stretch your thinking. When you know all the questions you're working on will have something to do with physics, you already have some sense for the context. What do we recommend? We recommend using the second method, of course.

The second method is to work through the questions arranged in a random order. Many Q&A resources offer comprehensive "practice tests." The extra challenge of not knowing, in advance, the subject of the next question generally helps you prepare more thoroughly and more closely matches the real testing situation for most exams. It forces you to pay attention more carefully to the presentation of the context of the question. When working through multiple-choice questions from within the same content area, an examinee is more prone to distracting thoughts that draw their focus away from the question itself; for example, "'B' can't be the answer to this question, it was the answer to the last three questions." Working across content areas and topics minimizes these unproductive thoughts. Working across topics exposes you to more material and affords the opportunity for you to compare and contrast facts and ideas, make associations, broaden your perspective, and think creatively in novel ways.

We must also offer a cautionary note about practicing with multiple-choice questions. As we previously mentioned, some students try to review as many questions as they can so that if they see a comparable question on the real exam they will already know the answer. Unfortunately, this is a source of needless mistakes, especially when the context of the question is important to selecting the best answer. As you answer practice questions, you form memory traces. These traces light up when you see a similar question on the real exam. When this recognition happens, you think "Aha! I've seen this before" and you answer it the same way as you did during the practice test, sometimes without even reading it through. The problem is that it's not the same question; it may have similar elements, but it is in fact a different question. Don't fall victim to mistaken identity.

Obtaining Feedback

In addition to learning content and expanding your appreciation of context, studying for standardized tests with multiple-choice questions offers you many additional opportunities for improvement. Possibly the most significant and valuable function of practice multiple-choice questions is the feedback they can provide. You can use this feedback to improve (1) the quality of your content knowledge, (2) your problem-solving abilities, and (3) your self-regulatory skills. However, being able to take advantage of this requires you to take action. No more Q&A drill sessions in which you just plow through question after question after question. You will need to plan your practice question sessions, time them, jot down notes while answering the practice questions, be methodical in your analysis of your performance, and reflect on the results of your analysis. We recommend the following strategy.

Q&A Feedback

To be productive, you will need some uninterrupted time to work, preferably in a quiet location. You should plan to set a pace of one question per minute on average, so if you have an hour available to you, plan to answer 60 questions. If you have 10 minutes, answer 10 questions. To get the most value out of this, follow the steps in the order in which we describe them.

1. Set a timer for the predetermined period of time. To be fully prepared for your upcoming exam, you need to train yourself to work at an average rate of one item per minute. Being able to maintain this pace, especially over a period of hours, will take practice. Practicing to answer questions in a timed environment will help you develop reading fluency (the ability to read quickly) and reading accuracy. An often-overlooked reason for examinees to fail standardized tests is not a lack of content knowledge or understanding, but a lack of ability to work effectively in a timed environment (Laatsch, 2009).
2. You will need paper to record all your answers and make some notations. This is true even if you are using a computer-based Q&A resource that keeps track of your answers electronically. You can answer the questions on the computer, but also note your answers on the sheet of paper. Number the paper with the number of questions you will be doing in this session.
3. Record each of your answers on the numbered sheet and make a notation next to each, indicating either (a) I know this (know), (b) I think I know this (think), or (c) This is an absolute guess

(guess). This information will be used to provide extremely important feedback.

4. After you've answered all the questions, *do not score them yet*; read the explanations without knowing if you got them right or wrong. We repeat—do not determine how many questions you got correct until you've read the explanations. If you selected the wrong answer, you are more likely to be defensive and try to come up with excuses as to why you got it wrong. It's better to read the explanation with an open mind (Brockkamp & Van Hout-Wolters, 2007; Crooks, 1988).

5. Determine how many, as well as which, questions you got right and wrong within each of the three categories: know, think, and guess (see Figure 9-5).

Step #5 is the point of this exercise. You need to gauge the accuracy of your metacognitive knowledge meter. When you are sure you know the answer, you want to get it right. If you guess and you get it wrong, it's OK. Obviously, it would be great to guess correctly too, but guessing incorrectly does not indicate a problem with your metacognitive skills. However, when you get a question wrong that you thought you knew, then you need to figure out why.

Whether you got something right or wrong when you only thought you knew the answer or you guessed means that you need to do some focused studying in that area—it points to a weakness in your content knowledge (see Figure 9-5). Getting something wrong that you were fairly confident you knew, on the other hand, presents a bigger challenge. You need to determine exactly why you missed the questions you thought you knew (see Chapter 9, Activity A). To do this, ask yourself a series of questions. Did I get this question wrong because I misread the stem or interrogatory of the question? Did I get the question wrong because I selected a correct answer, but not the best answer? Did I get this question wrong because I made a mistake in recording my answer selection? By answering these types of questions you can start to direct your subsequent studying.

If you were familiar with the information but had difficulty recalling specific details or making the proper associations—your challenge likely lies with the method you used to commit the content to memory (see Chapter 7 to review memory techniques and study skills). If you misread the stem of the question, you need to enhance your reading skills (see Chapters 8, 11, and 12). If you selected a correct answer, but

Figure 9-5

Breaking Down Practice MCQ Performance

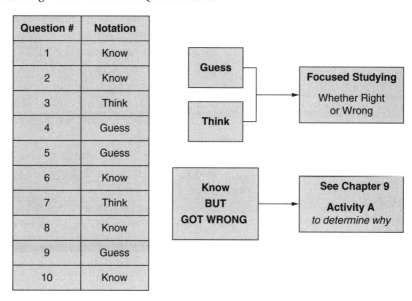

Question #	Notation
1	Know
2	Know
3	Think
4	Guess
5	Guess
6	Know
7	Think
8	Know
9	Guess
10	Know

not the best answer, you need to work on your test-taking skills (see Chapter 11 for a discussion of test-taking skills). If you knew the correct answer but wrote down an incorrect response, you need to focus on minimizing errors during the test (see Chapter 11).

GROUP STUDYING

In Chapter 5, we introduced the concept of learning styles and preferences, and briefly described the Myers–Briggs Type Indicator (MBTI). Just as your ability to remember is better when you associate new information to things you already know, so too is your ability to study and learn improved when you expand your learning style and step out of the comfort zone of your personality preferences.

You have the opportunity to expand your ability to learn when you become aware of your dominant and preferred learning style and take advantage of this knowledge to change your studying behaviors. For example, if you are a strong "Sensor" on the MBTI, you gain an advantage when you develop your "Intuitive" abilities; and vice versa (see Chapter 9, Activity B). Although we believe you can effectively study and learn to expand your skill set on your own, working with others has the potential to markedly advance your abilities.

If you have a person or persons in mind with whom you could study, it would be helpful for each of you to learn your MBTI. There are actually several online questionnaires to help you determine both your MBTI as well as your learning preferences. Simply type, "MBTI personality questionnaire" or "Learning styles questionnaire" into your search engine. There are advantages to working with people who have a different personality type.

Having more than one study partner can add value to your study session. Different people tend to have different learning styles and preferences. Adding members to a study group can provide a broader perspective—*if* you capitalize on and manage these differences, it can be a very positive experience. If the differences result in heated debate or off-topic discussions, then it is not such a good thing. The most important aspect of studying with other people is knowing what will maximize the benefit of this study approach while protecting one of your most important resources—time. Studying with other people has the potential to waste your time. It all depends on how you approach it.

To be most productive, study sessions need a PAL, which stands for: Plan–Agenda–Length. Whenever you meet with one or more people to study, you should have a plan that defines what you'd like to accomplish; an agenda that lists in some detail the topics you will cover; and a predetermined amount of time you will spend together studying. This will help everyone involved prepare for the session and, if you stick with your agenda, it will help keep the sessions on track.

The single biggest advantage of studying with a partner or in a small group is the exchange of ideas and the sharing of multiple perspectives (Michael, 2006). If everyone is motivated to learn and they arrive ready to have a discussion, ask questions, and provide explanations, then there is a lot that can be accomplished. Each person in the group could identify specific topics or concepts they found particularly challenging and take turns explaining what they know and understand. If none of you are sure, you can each look up some information and share what you have found. You can ask each other questions or even share the questions you have written and take each other's practice tests. When you answer the questions of a colleague, you test and expand your own understanding. Your study partner(s) can bring to your attention issues you may have overlooked or provide a new way of looking at things, and enhance your memory, recall, and ability to apply information in a broader context. There's really no limit to the possibilities, but it does take discipline to avoid some of the pitfalls.

Beware of escape syndrome. Sometimes, when people get together to study they don't bring a PAL. Without a plan or an agenda, the study session can quickly devolve into a gripe session. The study partners discuss the test, but they don't prepare for the test. It's not unusual for the conversation to shift to expressing emotions—fear, anxiety, frustration, and resentment. This phenomenon—directing time to talking about the test, not preparing for the test—is referred to as "escape syndrome." This is not at all productive and is best avoided entirely. If you can't rally the group back to the purpose of the session, it's best to cancel or postpone and go study on your own.

SUMMARY

By the time most students enter high school or college they have developed some basic study skills. Some people stop there. Those who tend to always perform in the upper percentiles continue to add new techniques to their repertoire and refine the old ones. These people practice . . . a lot, but not just any practice, they learn through deliberate practice.

This chapter presented methods to help you take your test-preparation to the next level by transforming your "what–what" thinking into "why and when" thinking. The next *why* questions you might ask yourself are, Why should I settle for just knowing about the ways higher-scoring students prepare for tests? Why would I not enhance *my* ability to do better on my next test? Why not change *my* behavior, starting now?

SECTION III SUMMARY AND NEXT STEPS

The take-away message from Section III—*Practicing Your Skills*—is that high performers have developed, through practice, a set of skills, behaviors, and study methods that have helped them to be successful. It's hard work, but you can do it, too.

The key is using what you have learned about memory, metacognition, and higher-order thinking to figure out how to advance to the next level of achievement. What will motivate you to put in the time and effort? What will help you change your behavior? How can you get better at self-regulation?

These chapters have offered numerous suggestions. Start by choosing one or two of the methods we described and practice them. Identify people around you who do things you wish you could do better, and ask them to help you. Once you have mastered one new skill set or technique, choose another, then another. Any given technique or skill won't work in all situations. The more options you have available, the more study techniques you can learn to use effectively, then efficiently, the higher your test scores will become.

The first three sections of this book were intended to guide your preparation for the exam and set the stage for the Section IV—*Executing Your Game Plan (Test Day)*. This next section will help you do your best on test day.

Before proceeding to Chapter 10, please reflect on the following questions:

- What was the primary take-away message for you from this chapter?
- What information will be the easiest for you to include in your exam preparation?

Be sure to complete the Chapter 9 Activities before starting to read Chapter 10.

CHAPTER 9 ACTIVITY A

Determining Why You Got Practice Multiple-Choice Questions WRONG

Your performance (score) on a practice examination can provide useful information. Your overall score offers some degree of insight into your breadth of content mastery, your preparedness for the sample of questions that you answered, how confident you might be about your state of preparedness, the amount of anxiety that you experienced during the session, and so on. Better insight can be gained through a purposeful analysis of your performance.

Chaplin (2007) provided a framework for question analysis that promotes the use of "active study" behaviors to encourage and improve higher-order thinking skills. The framework is divided into two activities. The first involves grouping the practice items into one of three categories based on the type of critical thinking required to determine the answer—knowledge based, application, or analysis. The second consists of looking for patterns that explain the reason that an item was answered incorrectly—misread stem or answer, knowledge deficit, or misconception.

By completing the following template for every missed question on a practice examination, you should be able to identify areas that you can work on to improve your test-taking and your ability to prepare for tests. If you identify a clear pattern that explains the majority of your missed questions, work to correct it as you prepare for and take subsequent practice tests.

By determining the reason that the question was missed—knowledge-based, application, or analysis—how can you minimize the likelihood that this will occur a second time? How can you prevent it from occurring in another area or on a subsequent test? Do the explanations provided offer some insight? What other explanations can you add?

Determine how you will apply this knowledge to guide your studying.

Table		
9–1	**Activity 1**	
Critical Thinking Skill Required	**Possible Explanation**	
Knowledge-based	1. Never saw this content before 2. Familiar with the content but could not recall enough 3. Didn't understand a word or phrase	
Application	1. Drew an incorrect conclusion 2. Selected a partially correct but not the best answer	
Analysis	1. Missed a key element in the stem 2. Misread the interrogatory 3. Missed a pattern	

CHAPTER 9 ACTIVITY B

Using MBTI to Guide Your Studying

The MBTI is an instrument that can be used to gain self-awareness. The dichotomous dimensions of the MBTI identify natural tendencies or preferences. Being aware of these preferences provides an opportunity to modify how you approach situations. Knowing how you would naturally approach a situation allows an opportunity to change (i.e., self-regulate) (Krause, 2003; Myers et al., 1998; Pelley & Dalley, 2008).

Sensors (S types) tend to focus on details and facts. They prefer to memorize and see the practical application of things. A primary goal is to achieve a "soundness" of understanding.

Intuitives (N types) tend to focus on the big picture. They prefer to self-direct their studying and prefer to find innovative applications

Table 9–2	Suggested Study Behaviors for the Four Mental Function Pairs
Mental Function Pair	**Suggestions for Studying**
ST	Avoid memorizing the information *Work from details to big picture/concepts* *Build chunks and patterns from the facts* Study in a structured area
SF	Avoid selective reading *Read from beginning to end* *Explain it to a colleague* Relate to the information
NT	Avoid looking for the big picture *Understand why* *Work from conclusion to details* Use more drills / repetition
NF	Avoid daydreaming *Create a plan/follow a routine* *Organize the material; compare and contrast details* Ask for feedback (and listen to it)

for information. A primary goal is to achieve a "quickness" of understanding. How might an S type benefit from thinking like an N type and vice versa?

Thinkers (T types) tend to be objective and impersonal. They prefer to focus on logic, using their left hemisphere to learn serially. They tend to note inconsistencies in information.

Feelers (F types) tend to perceive things as worthwhile or not. They prefer to focus on value, using their right hemisphere to learn randomly. They prefer to maintain harmony. How might a T type benefit from thinking like an F type and vice versa?

CHAPTER 9 ACTIVITY C

Using Creative Thinking

Becoming most efficient in the process of exam preparation often benefits from the use of creative thinking. Many individuals experience blocks during examination preparation that slows or stops learning. Creative thinking can help you overcome or eliminate these blocks.

Consider the times when your mind wanders and you have particular trouble staying in the here and now. Identify the time or times when efforts to return to studying were particularly difficult and your mind wandered repeatedly. There are strategies that you can use to work through these blocks and return to the here and now. Recall the most recent time when a block seemed overwhelming and develop a plan to work around the block using the following strategies:

1. Rethinking
   a. Consider new reasons why the block occurred and brainstorm for ideas.
   b. Consider the process of overcoming the block as a challenge that can be conquered.
2. Visualization
   a. You have identified the problem or sources for the problem and can now visualize all of the factors influencing and producing the block.
   b. Remember it's a challenge that can be solved.

3. Combinations
    a. There may not be one solution but rather many factors that may need multiple actions.
    b. Make connections and establish new relationships as needed.
4. Think in extremes
    a. Some blocks require extensive revisions in your plans for success.
    b. Don't be afraid to make a major change if needed.

Remember that some long-standing losing streaks in sports are broken only after an entirely new management team is in place with a new game plan.

Part

2

Taking Your Test (Applying Test-Taking Skills)

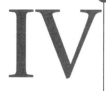
IV

Executing Your Game Plan (Test Day)

IT'S TIME TO SHOW WHAT YOU KNOW!

On the very first page of the introduction to this book we stated that high examination scores are the result of two factors: (1) optimal preparation before the test and (2) optimal performance during the test. Let's suppose you've followed our advice in the first three sections: (I) *Understanding Your Opponent* (The Test), (II) *Developing Your TEAMS*, and (III) *Practicing Your Skills*. You have developed test-wiseness. Now it's time to develop your test-taking skills. That's what this section is about: executing your game plan on test day.

Here's where you pull it all together. Section IV covers three essential topics for optimal performance during the exam: (1) managing the time clock, (2) maximizing your points, and (3) minimizing test anxiety. It's about reaching your potential.

Adequate preparation—both the right kind and the right amount—is necessary to good performance, but it is not sufficient. Getting a high test score isn't just about knowledge, memory, and problem-solving skills. In fact, there are people who are so good at taking tests they can outperform more knowledgeable test-takers. You may know someone like that; it can be very frustrating to someone who has studied long and hard. The good news is that this is a learnable set of skills.

Chapter 10

Managing the Time Clock

People who have otherwise prepared well for a standardized exam can get tripped up from having to work under the pressure of time constraints. There are essentially three factors that account for this: stress, pace, and fatigue. All exams have time limits; however, standardized tests often require you to work at a faster rate—answer more questions per given unit of time—than the typical classroom exam, generally in the neighborhood of one question per minute. People often mentally collapse under the added stress caused by this increased pace. Therefore, you must prepare for it through practice and planning. Furthermore, most standardized exams require you to maintain a faster rate of answering questions over a significantly greater span of time than a typical classroom exam, usually between 4 and 8 hours. This too can take some getting used to, but it is also something you can prepare for.

Think of the marathon runner who not only trains to improve distance and speed, but also pace and stamina. Runners have a time goal and they work on being able to meet it without burning themselves out. It's part of their training and they think about it beforehand. In other words, they develop and practice a strategy, which they can execute on the day of the big race.

In Chapter 9 we recommended that you practice answering questions from your Q&A resources using a time allocation of approximately one minute per item. If you practice using that approach, you will be much better prepared to manage the time clock, and you will be less likely to find yourself running out of time before you've completed the exam. However, there's even more you can do than simply time yourself while answering practice questions. This chapter will help you understand what to expect and how to be successful while working in an unusually stressful, timed environment.

- How can you maintain a good pace when you're feeling the pressure?
- What techniques can help you work more quickly without reducing your effectiveness?
- What can you do to add points to your score while reducing the likelihood that you will commit avoidable errors that occur more often when challenged to work under time constraints?
- How can you prepare for and cope with fatigue that results from such a long test?

Answers to these questions can be found in the pages that follow.

WORKING IN A TIMED ENVIRONMENT: KEYS TO SUCCESS

Success Key #1: Have a Plan Before You Get There

If you're a worrier and prone to anxiety, knowing as much as possible about what to expect and having a detailed, concrete plan will go a long way toward alleviating some of the anxiety associated with fear of the unknown. As a bonus, planning ahead will reduce the likelihood of something actually going terribly wrong on the day of the exam. There's nothing more challenging than working at an uncomfortable pace, except possibly doing so when you've already experienced a setback, such as getting to the testing center only to find that you forgot your ID or that they won't let you in wearing your baggy shirt and sweatpants.

This refers back to the notion of getting to know your opponent. You should become well acquainted with the rules of the exam and the testing center.

- Do you need one or two forms of picture ID to check in?
- What are you allowed to bring in with you? Depending on what you're allowed to bring with you to the testing center, you might consider creating a self-care kit containing medicine for headaches or stomachaches and snacks.
- Will there be a locker in which you can keep your personal items? If not, you will want to think twice before bringing your cell phone or other electronic device because it is almost a sure thing that you will not be allowed to bring these into the actual testing room with you.
- Are there any restrictions on clothing, such as a no-hat policy (very likely)? Some centers also do not allow loose clothing or jackets to be worn in the testing room.
- Can you wear earplugs (probably not)?
- Can you wear a watch? If so, then you should.
- Is there a drinking fountain or vending machine available?
- Can you have bottled water in the testing room?
- How long is the exam?
- How many questions are there?
- How is the day broken up?
- How many breaks do you get?

You will also want to make sure you know where the testing center is located and what driving route you will take to get there. You might even want to have driven the route beforehand, if possible, and identified a backup route in case of bad traffic. If you live over two hours from the testing center and you have an early morning exam, you might want to consider staying in a nearby hotel the night before.

There is a great deal to learn and plan for before your test day arrives. Optimal execution requires avoiding, to the best of your ability, the chance of being blindsided by something unexpected. Don't contribute to the pressure of the day by not knowing what to expect.

Success Key #2: Arrive at the Testing Center 45 Minutes Early

The last thing you want is to arrive late to the testing center, if for no other reason than they might turn you away and you will forfeit the exam fee. The second to last thing you want is to arrive just moments before the scheduled start time. This added stress can and should be avoided. If your personality is such that you tend to fly by the seat of your pants with little care as to whether you're on time to scheduled events, this is definitely one of those life moments (job interviews are another) when your natural inclinations and preferences seriously put you at a disadvantage.

You should plan to arrive at least 45 minutes prior to the scheduled start of your test. If you will be driving to your testing site, determine the commute time to the location. If it will take less than 60 minutes, give yourself an additional 30 minutes. If the commute time is more than 60 minutes, give yourself an additional hour. In other words, anticipate delays, plan accordingly, and leave extra early.

When you arrive at the testing site, you will need to check in. It is common to require one or more pieces of picture identification to gain entrance to a national standardized test. Be sure you know what you need to bring. Don't be surprised if you are also fingerprinted during the check-in process.

After check-in, proceed to the testing area, but before you enter, locate the restrooms, vending machines, and drinking fountains. Once in the testing area, ask if there is a white board or pencil and paper that you can use during the exam. Familiarize yourself with the layout of your testing station. If the exam is computerized, use the allotted time to complete the tutorial so you are aware of the features of the software being used. Some exam websites include the tutorial. If so, this is something else you should consider doing before test day.

Pay attention to the behavioral and procedural expectations for each stage of the testing process: beginning, throughout, and end of the test. Know if it's acceptable to leave the testing area—and if so, under what circumstances? What is the procedure? Where is the proctor located? Be sure you know what you can and can't do. Testing centers and agencies monitor for irregular behavior. Know the regulations regarding acceptable behavior. This is no time to express your antiauthority, rebel-with-or-without-a-cause attitude; you have too much to lose. You do not want to end your exam only to learn that it will not be scored or that you are being sanctioned for some questionable activity. Can we say, "Know the policies and rules of the testing agency and testing site" one more time to be sure you know how important this is?

We're pretty sure that you're feeling a little overwhelmed right now. Who knew there was so much else to know and do in order to excel on a standardized test? Answer: you do…now! It's not as overwhelming as it seems if you take it one step at a time.

In summary—know the rules, arrive early, get the lay of the land, settle in, and know the rules!

Success Key #3: Pace Yourself

The goal of pacing is to work quickly enough that you don't run out of time, but not so fast that you rush and sacrifice accuracy. There's no need to panic; the time allotted for a standardized test is sufficient especially if you've done some planning and preparation beforehand. The clock is not your enemy.

Exam Structure

As we mentioned in Success Key #1, you want to do some research beforehand. In terms of managing the time clock, here are some questions you should have answered:

- How long is the exam? Four hours? Eight hours?
- How is the time divided up over the course of the entire exam? How many sections or question blocks are there? How much time is allocated per block? How many questions per block?
- Are you given any breaks? How many? How long? Do the breaks count against your time?
- Can you proceed through the sections at your own pace? If a section takes you longer than the allotted time are you forced to move on even if you haven't finished? If you are making your way more quickly through the questions, must you wait to move on to the next section until a certain period of time has elapsed?
- Can you go back to a section once you've exited it, or is the section closed as soon as you proceed to the next section?

Time per Question

Once you know how much time you have and how many questions there are, you need to do some simple arithmetic so you can develop a time-use plan. For example, if there are 50 questions per one-hour block, then you have 1.2 minutes or 72 seconds per question. However, we recommend that you factor in one other variable: leaving yourself some time at the end to go back to the questions you've flagged and check your work. If you allot 10 minutes at the end of each question block for this, then the calculation becomes 50 questions per 50 minutes, or one question per minute. Obviously some questions will take more time, some will take less; one minute per question is an average. If you obtain this information early enough, you can practice your plan while you're doing practice questions. Practice will help the pace become second-nature to you so you are more likely to stick to it on test day even when the pressure is on.

Question Sequence

Some computerized tests allow you to complete the questions in any order. We suggest that for any type of exam, you complete them sequentially, in the order that they appear. Even if you don't know the answer to a question, answer it anyway. We are not aware of any common standardized exam that still has a penalty for wrong answers.

Most tests allow you to mark or "flag" the questions you would like to return to later. By answering each question when you read it, and flagging the ones you're unsure of, you eliminate the possibility of accidentally leaving a question unanswered (we discuss effective guessing techniques in the next chapter). If you don't answer a question, you will definitely not get it right, so it's better to guess than to skip. Flagging questions for review will give you the opportunity to rethink and possibly change your answer before you move on to the next section (we discuss changing answers in the next chapter).

Difficult Questions

One tricky aspect of managing the time clock is figuring out how much time to spend puzzling through the tough questions. People often make the mistake of letting a real stumper throw their timing way off, potentially causing them to run out of time.

We suggest you develop a plan for difficult questions, and practice your plan while you're preparing for the test—again, a good use of practice questions. For starters, use your metacognitive knowledge to gauge whether the question content is something for which you have any significant knowledge—are you close to getting it or is nothing coming to you at all? If you have absolutely no clue, simply make a random guess and move on immediately—flag it if you must, but don't spend any time on it. If you're close, but struggling, use the full minute to rule out the options that are obviously wrong, then make your best guess, flag it, and move on.

Time flies when you're freaking out, so it is worthwhile to remind yourself that standardized tests contain a percentage of pilot items; tell yourself that this is one of them and move on. Be aware that it is not entirely unusual for test-takers to encounter a whole string of difficult questions. Treat each one in the manner we outlined above—tests are taken one question at a time. Panic will only make matters much worse.

There are several good reasons to leave a difficult question behind. (1) Statistically, you are more likely to get them wrong anyway, so don't waste the time. (2) Sometimes when you get stuck in your thinking, you need to "step away" from it for a bit—something might come to you later. (3) There might be a clue in a later question. (4) If you use too much time, you will have to rush through other questions that would have been easier if you had enough time.

Be Mindful of the Time

We do not advocate that you become a clock watcher who is preoccupied with how much time you have left. However, you do need to have a general level of awareness of the amount of time remaining in each section, so that you can maintain the pace you predetermined.

Let's continue to work with our example of 50 questions per hour. When you reach the halfway point—30 minutes into the section—you should have answered at least 25 of the items. If you have answered fewer than 20 you need to pick up the pace. If you have answered more than 30, you might want to slow down a bit to ensure you are reading accurately. It's not a race and there's no prize for finishing first. You might also want to glance at a clock or your watch when you encounter a particularly difficult question so that you do not spend too much time working on it.

Success Key #4: Check Your Work

After all the time, effort, and emotion you have invested into preparing for the test, the last thing that you want to do is make a careless error, which reduces your score. Prior to exiting any section of the test be sure to verify the accuracy of your work. Be sure you have answered all of the questions. Review all flagged questions. If taking a pencil-and-paper exam, make sure you have accurately transferred all of your answers to the answer sheet. We will return to the topic of error avoidance in Chapter 11.

Success Key #5: Maintain Your Stamina

There are actually several things you can do to minimize mental and physical fatigue on test day:

- Incorporate a stamina-increasing practice into your exam preparation process. Once a week prior to your exam, take a long, timed practice exam. For example, every Saturday morning, set aside 4 hours to complete 200 questions.
- Get plenty of sleep—at least 7 hours—the night before your exam, and preferably don't do any studying the day before the test. Absolutely do not stay up all night cramming. There is nothing you can learn that will be worth the performance drop you will have from lack of sleep. Even if you feel you will do nothing but toss and turn, it is likely you will take a series of micronaps throughout the night, and in any case, you will be more rested by lying in bed than if you stay up all night doing something.
- Eat a healthy breakfast—complex carbohydrates and light protein.
- Take all the breaks that are available to you.
- If the exam has both a morning and an afternoon session, eat a light lunch in between—complex carbohydrates and light protein. Avoid simple sugars—you might get an energy boost but you are also likely to experience a crash.
- Use caffeine sparingly during the days leading up to the exam. If you need a pick-me-up on exam day, don't overdo it, and don't use caffeine unless you know how your body and mind react to it.
- Stay hydrated as best as you can. Dehydration can cause headaches and fatigue. You will probably not be able to bring water into the testing room with you; however, try to drink a little bit

during each break. Don't drink so much that you have to use the bathroom frequently.

- Most people experience an afternoon slump. During the afternoon session, you might need to take more frequent mental breaks. Pause for 30 seconds to close your eyes and stretch your neck muscles by gently bending your neck side to side as though you're trying to touch your ear to your shoulder.
- If you're taking a computerized exam, eye fatigue will also be an issue. Periodically look away from the computer and try to focus on a faraway object. Use your best judgment regarding where to look—you don't want it to look like you are trying to cheat.

Checklist

√ Learn about the testing center facilities and rules as to what you can and cannot bring with you.

√ Plan your driving route and have an alternative route (drive it once beforehand if you live close enough to the testing center).

√ If you live far from the center (>2 hours), consider spending the night in a hotel nearby.

√ Set your alarm clock and have a backup alarm (or schedule a wake-up call).

√ The night before lay out everything needed for test day, including comfortable clothing, two forms of picture ID, snacks, medicine for headache or stomachache, and watch.

√ Leave from home earlier than seems necessary in case there is a traffic jam or train delay.

√ Arrive early at the test center, check in, and get settled in.

Take some deep breaths and get ready to rock that test.

SUMMARY

For some examinees, one of the major challenges associated with standardized tests is working under a time crunch. Don't let this be one of your challenges. As with most things in life, the more knowledge you have and the more planning you do, the better off you'll be. As we discussed in Section I of this book, getting to know your opponent is an important part of the exam preparation process. This includes learning what to expect on exam day. Furthermore, there are things you can actually do before the exam to make the day less stressful.

We proposed five keys to successfully managing the time clock. (1) Have a plan before you get there. (2) Arrive at the testing center 45 minutes early. (3) Pace yourself. (4) Check your work. (5) Maintain your stamina.

As we have stated so many times throughout this book, knowing and doing are not the same. If you already knew the information we have presented, we have reinforced its importance. If you did not know these things, you know them now. Only you can decide what you will do. In Chapter 11 we present more thoughts on things you need to know and do. We hope you do them.

Before proceeding to Chapter 11, please reflect on the following questions:

- What was the primary take-away message for you from this chapter?
- What information will be the easiest for you to include in your exam preparation?

Be sure to complete the Chapter 10 Activity before starting to read Chapter 11.

CHAPTER 10 ACTIVITY

Working Efficiently in a Timed Environment

Chapter 10—*Managing the Time Clock*—presented several methods to facilitate your ability to work efficiently during your test without compromising your effectiveness. Respond to the items below to reinforce your planning and thinking about how you will augment your capacity to answer questions in a timed environment.

Table	
10–1	**Activity 1**

a. What did I learn about the test format from the test website?

b. What will I do to ensure that I arrive at my testing site early?

c. Based on my testing session timeframe, when do I need to be halfway done?

d. How much time will I allocate to difficult or complex questions?

e. What safeguards will I use to avoid making careless and/or needless errors?

Chapter

11 | Maximizing Your Points

We'd be very surprised if you haven't already answered many multiple-choice questions in your life. In fact, it's likely you've answered most of them correctly, but how many did you get wrong that you could have or should have answered correctly? Why did this happen, and are there ways you can minimize the frequency of this occurrence in the future?

Working under the pressure of a perceived time crunch increases the likelihood of making preventable errors that result from such behaviors as skimming through the question, overlooking or misinterpreting an essential piece of information, failing to use a high-probability approach to guessing, changing right answers to wrong answers, and mismarking answers when recording your answer selection. Regardless of your time and efforts invested to this point, no matter how well prepared you might be, committing these types of errors can dramatically lower your score. High-scoring individuals rarely make these kinds of avoidable mistakes. It has been reported that using effective test-taking skills can increase a test score by more than ten percentile points (Bangert-Drowns, Kulik, & Kulik, 1983).

HOW CAN YOU IMPROVE YOUR TEST-TAKING SKILLS?

To help you understand why errors are made and what you can do to avoid them, we've divided this chapter into five sections: (1) avoiding reading and interpretation errors, (2) narrowing the options, (3) best practices when guessing, (4) changing answers, and (5) avoiding careless errors.

Avoiding Reading and Interpretation Errors

Let's begin by reiterating some concepts related to memory that we introduced in Chapter 7. Recall that sensory information enters your short-term memory (STM), which processes this large volume of unorganized information into larger, more manageable chunks. Your working memory (WM), a component of STM, can hold about seven of these chunks for a period of time less than a minute.

Why does this matter? Think about it this way: as you read a test question, the words enter your brain as sensory information, and this goes into your WM. At the same time, the information you're reading functions to provide memory cues for associated information you have stored in your long-term memory (LTM)—you recognize the words, you know what they mean, you might recall an episode in which you first learned that information, you think about how the information is all related together. To answer the question, some of the information stored in your LTM is pulled back into WM and combined with the current influx of sensory information. Any other thoughts or sensations you are experiencing at the moment—worry about failing, negative thoughts about your ability, sensations of discomfort, sounds coming from all around you—also enter into this mix, and all of it is competing for the same limited space. When you think about it that way, it's amazing we can function at all, but the brain is an amazing processing organ, and there's a lot more going on than we have described (or even understand).

You may recall that we advised you to not underestimate the importance of STM in your ability to problem-solve. The limited capacity and duration of STM can lead to numerous errors when reading, interpreting, and answering test questions. Furthermore, human thought processes are far from perfectly logical, and we are prone to a multitude of cognitive biases when making decisions. Being aware of some of the more common of these can help you avoid them.

Mental Mistakes

The first step in preparing to answer a question is to understand what the question is asking. Seems simple enough, right? Recall that many questions begin with a stem—a series of sentences that frame the problem. You want to be sure that you draw the appropriate conclusions from the question stem. If you fail to develop an accurate representation of the question in your working memory, you will likely choose a wrong answer.

Long questions—those consisting of more than a sentence or two— are more daunting to understand and process and for good reason. These questions not only tax our stored knowledge in LTM, but they also bump up against the limits of our STM capacity. Apart from simply not knowing the information required to answer the question (lacking content knowledge), the two primary reasons for selecting the wrong answer are reading errors and cognitive biases.

Reading Errors

Reading errors tend to occur when you try to read too quickly, skim the question, lack focus, or overlook details. The general solution is to read each question and all of the options carefully and make sure you understand what is being asked. Don't assume you "get it" before you've read the entire question stem. Identify the critical information. Pay attention to not only the key content information (e.g., the facts presented, but also the parts of speech, such as verbs, adverbs, conjunctions, prepositions, and adjectives—these are important). Look for words that qualify or add specificity to factual statements. Look for thought-shifting words such as but, however, despite, and except—these words can make the difference between a right and wrong answer.

Overlooking or intentionally ignoring pertinent information is a surefire way to select the wrong answer. The information contained within the question stem is there to help you select the correct answer. Don't dismiss details; they're there for a reason. Pay attention to the particulars presented. For example: the event occurred at 1:00 a.m. EST on December 22, 2011, the person was a 25-year-old female, and the room was rectangular in shape and was twice as long as it was wide. Questions on standardized exams do not contain "filler information"; the details are not there to mislead you. That's not to say a skilled question writer won't throw in a word or two that could lead a less knowledgeable or less skilled test-taker in the wrong direction or cause them to jump to a premature conclusion. When information in the question stem seems misleading, it is because either you have misunderstood it or you have a superficial understanding of the concepts being tested. The information in the question stem is directing you to see a pattern and you can't afford to miss it.

One of the best ways to develop an accurate appreciation of the test question is to analyze the information as it is presented, making predictions as you go. As each new piece of information is revealed, actively compare and contrast the answer possibilities that come to mind. As you continue to read the question ask yourself, does it support, refute, or have no impact on what I am thinking?

Faulty reasoning or faulty logic occurs when your conclusion is not supported by the facts as they've been presented. The main types of faulty reasoning likely to influence your answer selection are circular reasoning (e.g., this is the best answer because I think it's the best answer), overgeneralization (i.e., thinking in absolutes—this is always/never true), false causality (e.g., because A came after B, B must have caused A), oversimplification (i.e., assuming a single cause when, in fact, there are many), and making assumptions that are not true (e.g., they are factually incorrect or based on your opinion). It is important that your rationale for selecting the answer be based on sound reasoning.

The interrogatory of a question is the part that poses the challenge to you—the part that actually "asks the question." This is usually the last sentence. If you misread or don't understand the question being asked, even if you interpreted all elements of the stem correctly you can still select the wrong answer to the question. You need to pay attention to the word choice in the interrogatory. Is the interrogatory asking: What's the *most likely* cause of X? or What's the *most common* cause of X? There's a difference, and these word choices matter. Once you've made your answer selection, read the interrogatory again to make sure you have in fact answered the question.

Cognitive Biases

Humans have many, many cognitive biases that can impact negatively on the accuracy of our decision-making processes (Croskerry, 2003; Kempainen, Migeon, & Wolf, 2003). One of the interesting facets of our thinking is that when a lot of information is presented sequentially, our recall of it is influenced by its relative position in the sequence. This is called the "serial position effect." This bias is particularly problematic with longer questions. Each portion of the question—beginning, middle, end—has the potential to unduly influence the decision-making process leading to the wrong answer selection.

The *primacy effect* refers to the bias in which information at the beginning of the question is better recalled, which can result in neglecting to consider information provided in the rest of the question when selecting your answer. When the bias is in favor of information toward the end of the question it is known as the *recency effect*. If you've ever seen the movie, *A Fish Called Wanda*, you might recall that Wanda's bank-robbing, knife-wielding brother Otto suffered from this type of cognitive bias. Whenever he was presented with a sequence of steps in a plan, he would ask, "What was the middle thing?" Depending on the length of the question, the middle portion can contain a significant amount of valuable information and detail that you do not want to ignore.

To try to minimize the impact of the serial position effect, refer back to the question when making your final answer selection. Also, try to encapsulate the key points of the question by jotting down brief notes on the whiteboard or paper that was supplied to you for use during the exam.

Premature closure is another form of cognitive bias in which you draw your conclusion before you have read and analyzed all of the available information. It's OK to be thinking of the possible answer to the question as you're reading it. In fact, we recommend you do; however, it's important that you don't make your *final* selection before you've finished reading the question. It's also important that you do not discount any of the information provided, especially if it challenges your initial impression. This also holds true with the options—read all of them even if you think you already know the answer. If what you thought was the correct answer is among the options, then this is *most likely* the correct answer. However, before you make your final selection, read all the options and benchmark them against your first choice. Make sure the answer you've selected is not just a correct answer; make sure it's the *best* answer.

Narrowing the Options

The advantage of a multiple-choice exam over an essay exam is that the correct answer is right there in front of you. Your job is to select it, not recall it from memory or create it entirely on your own. If you possess the appropriate level of knowledge and you understand the interrogatory, it's generally easy to select the best answer. What if you can't, however? Sometimes you can only rule out wrong answers. Do this. Eliminate as many options as possible; this will increase the probability of making the correct choice. Once you have narrowed your options, reread the question again. Sometimes rereading the question with a new frame of mind will allow you to see something you missed before. Don't just keep staring at the options waiting for one to light up.

For many questions, each option should be treated like a true–false statement. As you read each option, keep track, by marking on the whiteboard or paper, which options are true and which are false. Don't mistake a true statement for a correct answer. Questions, especially higher-order questions on standardized exams, might include several options that are "correct." You need to select the "best" option, which means the option that best fits with the information in the question stem and that actually answers the question posed in the interrogatory. When in doubt, reread the question.

Best Practices When Guessing

Guessing well is a skill that elite test-takers have mastered. We certainly don't advocate guessing in place of using your knowledge and problem-solving skills to select an answer. That being said, there are times, as you no doubt already know based on your own experience, when you read a question and have absolutely no idea what the question is about; you know nothing about the subject at all. It is useful in these moments to remember that the correct answer is among the five options. You have a choice: (1) take a purely random guess or (2) use "clues" in the question to increase your probability of guessing correctly. Skilled test-takers can often identify—and use to their advantage—these clues (Evans, 1984). If guessing is your only alternative, wouldn't it be a good idea to "guess best"? A major caveat to the following "best practices" is that they tend to rely on sloppy test writing. For most standardized exams, the questions have been so thoroughly vetted that they do not provide the clues described as follows, which is why these practices should be used only when guessing is your last resort.

Practice #1: The General Alternative

Examine the options for their degree of specificity. Select the more general option (Dolly & Williams, 1986; Sarnacki, 1979). If more than one option is fairly general, use best practice #9 to select among the general options.

Practice #2: Avoid Absolutes

Identify the adjectives each option includes. Correct responses typically do not include absolute statements (always, never, must, none, only). Select an option containing adjectives that permit exceptions (seldom, usually, often, perhaps) (Milman, Bishop, & Ebel, 1965, cited in Dolly & Williams, 1986; Sarnacki, 1979). If more than one option allows exceptions, again use best practice #9.

Practice #3: Middle of the Range

When presented with a series of numerical options, the correct response is often in the middle of the range, not at either extreme (Milman et al., 1965).

Practice #4: The Deductive Approach (Convergence Strategy)

If each of the options represents a set of variables, first identify all of the variables presented in all of the options. Next, count the number of times each variable is included in any of the options. Then, select as your final answer the one option that contains the set of variables that were included the greatest number of times in all of the options (Smith, 1982, cited in Dolly & Williams, 1986; Sarnacki, 1979).

Practice #5: The Clang Association

If a word or phrase that appears in the question stem is repeated exactly or very similarly to one of the options, select that option (Diamond & Evans, 1972 cited in Dolly & Williams, 1986; Sarnacki, 1979).

Practice #6: Similar and Opposite Alternatives

Examine the options for those that are the same or the opposite. If two options mean essentially the same thing, and for all intents and purposes you cannot distinguish between them, then the correct response is not likely to be one of them. The correct response is often one of two opposite alternatives (Millman, 1969, cited in Dolly & Williams, 1986; Sarnacki, 1979).

Practice #7: Select the Longest Alternative

Sometimes, without being aware of it, the exam writer includes more information in the correct response. If one of the five options is disproportionately longer than the others, select it (Chase, 1964 cited in Dolly & Williams, 1986; Sarnacki, 1979).

Practice #8: Avoid Question–Answer Grammar Disagreement

The question and options should be in grammatical agreement—an interrogatory that is singular should not be completed with a plural option; an interrogatory that is plural should not be completed with a singular option (Board & Whitney, 1972, cited in Dolly & Williams, 1986; Sarnacki, 1979). This is more likely to assist you in ruling out an incorrect response.

Practice #9: Making a Random Guess

When all else has truly failed, and you've ruled out as many options as you can, you should have a predetermined strategy that makes it easy to quickly take a random guess. We don't suggest looking at your previous answers and guessing based on some perceived pattern or selecting a specific letter because you haven't used it in a while. It's not random enough, and it takes too much thought and time. Some people always choose the same option, such as "C," when they're guessing, but what if you've already ruled that option out. Another method, and the one we suggest, is to always select the first option remaining after you've done your best to rule out as many as possible. If you haven't ruled out any options, pick A. If you've ruled out A, pick B. If you've ruled out A and B, pick C, and so on.

Practice #10: Guess Only as a Last Resort!

It is always best to use knowledge and reasoning to select the best answer and to rule out as many options as possible. Only use guessing techniques as a last resort, and *never* talk yourself out of an educated guess in lieu of one of the foregoing practices.

Changing Answers

Well-intentioned individuals have admonished many of us to "never change your first answer." However, this advice is not borne out of research. Each time you change an answer, there are three possible outcomes: wrong to right, right to wrong, or wrong to wrong. Results of studies showed that approximately 55% of answers were changed *from wrong to right*—the preferred direction—and that the remainder was fairly evenly divided between the other two possibilities (Benjamin, Cavell, & Shallenberger, 1984; Kruger, Wirtz, & Miller, 2005).

The question is not should you or shouldn't you change your first answer; the question is under what conditions should you. Don't change your first answer based on low self-confidence (i.e., second-guessing). Don't change a first guess to a second guess. On a five-option question (choices A–E), you have a 20% chance that your first guess will be correct. If your first guess was correct and you change it, the probability that you will have changed your right answer to a wrong answer is 100%. If your first guess was wrong and you change it, the probability that you will change it to the correct answer is 25% (you have four options to choose from and one of those four is correct), *but* the probability that you will change your first wrong guess to a second wrong guess is 75% (you have four options remaining and three of the four are wrong). So, if you guessed the first time, stick with it.

Also, don't change your first answer because you're overthinking the question—take the question at face value.

UNDER WHAT CONDITIONS SHOULD YOU CHANGE YOUR ANSWER?

Do change your first answer if you have an epiphany—a sudden realization that gives you insight—during the test and (1) you now realize your first guess was wrong, and (2) you now know what the correct answer is. How might you have an epiphany? Perhaps you read a question later in the test that stimulates a thought that brings information to your working memory that wasn't accessible earlier. Or perhaps some bit of knowledge just pops into your head for no apparent reason. We've all had that experience in which some memory we were trying to dredge up didn't come to us until after we'd stopped trying. Epiphanies are rare, but when they do occur take advantage of them. The only other instance in which it is a good idea to rethink your first guess is if upon rereading the question you realize you misread it the first time. In these two cases—epiphanies and first-time misreading—there is a high probability you will change a wrong answer to a correct answer.

> **Critical Comment:** Don't confuse a second hunch or guess with an epiphany!

Avoiding Careless Errors

Careless errors, such as mismarking your answer selection or inadvertently skipping a question, result from being distracted, for example, by worry thoughts, by being overly tired, or from trying to go too quickly. Make sure you get enough sleep the night before the exam, slow down, and check your work.

SUMMARY

You studied for a long time in preparation for the exam, and you want your score to reflect your effort and your knowledge. To assist you in achieving this goal, Chapter 11 addressed five ways to maximize your points on the exam: (1) avoiding reading and interpretation errors, (2) narrowing the options, (3) using best practices when guessing, (4) changing answers, and (5) avoiding careless errors.

Humans are prone to mistakes, especially when the pressure is on; nevertheless, by becoming aware of the more common types of errors and what causes them, you can develop a plan to help you avoid them. In addition, there are things you can do to help you narrow down the options when selecting your answer and there are techniques that can help you make a good guess, when guessing is your only option. Just as you can improve your ability to manage the time clock through planning and practice, you can also practice maximizing your points while doing practice questions in preparation for the exam.

Before proceeding to Chapter 12, please reflect on the following questions:

- What was the primary take-away message for you from this chapter?
- What information will be the easiest for you to include in your exam preparation?

Be sure to complete the Chapter 11 Activity before starting to read Chapter 12.

CHAPTER 11 ACTIVITY

Working Effectively in a Timed Environment

Chapter 11—*Maximizing Your Points*—made you aware that examinees with well-developed test-taking skills achieve higher test scores than equally well-prepared examinees without that skill set. Responding to the following items will help you further develop and hone your test-taking skills.

Table	
11–1	**Activity 1**

a. List five characteristics that help examinees avoid errors that reduce scores.

b. What techniques will you use to increase the probability of selecting the best answer?

c. When guessing is your only option, what methods help you "guess best"?

d. List three cognitive biases and ways to reduce their occurrence.

e. When should you change an answer on your test?

Chapter 12

Minimizing Test Anxiety

"Where did they get these questions?"
"Am I just not smart enough to pass this examination?"
"What will happen to me if I fail?"
"Will I be able to finish the exam if there are too many questions on topics I don't know?"

An excessive level of concern about test performance often manifests itself in the form of test anxiety. Researchers have established that test anxiety has been significantly increasing in our society over the past 20 years to the point of existing at high levels among persons taking standardized tests (Chapell, Blanding, Silverstein, & Gubi, 2005). Test anxiety can have a detrimental effect on examination performance as well on personal feelings in the postexamination period. Failure or low performance on tests can promote a heightened sense of self-doubt and a loss of identity. Although test anxiety can block desired outcomes on standardized examinations, the good news is that there are a variety of intervention options that are highly effective. The key is to identify and understand the specifics of test anxiety so that the best strategy for intervention can be employed. It has been demonstrated that the most effective intervention strategies for test anxiety are those using a combination of techniques geared to individual needs.

This chapter presents three steps to cope with and minimize test anxiety:

1. Recognizing the signs and effects of test anxiety
2. Understanding the mechanisms underlying test anxiety
3. Overcoming test anxiety through interventions

STEP 1: RECOGNIZING THE SIGNS AND EFFECTS OF TEST ANXIETY

Experiencing anxiety can be an aversive emotional event that usually motivates a person to get away from the anxiety-provoking situation. Anxiety can be identified in a number of ways including through subjective reports of feeling tense or fearful, an array of physiological signs of arousal, an increased sense of danger, avoidance behaviors, trying to flee a situation, and cognitive impairments (Ergene, 2003). Anxiety in itself is not necessarily detrimental to test performance. In fact moderate levels of anxiety have been found to be beneficial toward achievement of maximal examination outcomes. For the test-taker, anxiety becomes problematic when it is either unnecessarily low or high. This relationship of anxiety level to test performance is commonly portrayed as an inverted U shape with the beneficial moderate level of anxiety at the top of the inverted U shape. The two ends of the curve indicating low and high anxiety indicates low test performance (Weber & Bizer, 2005).

It is important to monitor one's level of anxiety related to taking standardized tests in order to maintain a moderate amount that promotes beneficial preparatory activities. However, it is also important to be cognizant of the fact that stressful life experiences in all areas of one's functioning can have a cumulative effect and increase overall levels of anxiety that could then manifest at a detrimental level of test anxiety. A general tip on managing test anxiety is to keep overall life stressors to a minimum and maintain a healthful lifestyle when preparing to complete a standardized test.

At the side of the inverted U-shaped curve where anxiety is low, the test performance is typically low as well. Persons with low levels of anxiety usually do not begin studying far enough in advance to succeed on tests, employ poor study habits, review material in an unorganized and haphazard fashion, lack of sense of urgency about the test, or do not perceive a need to study for the examination. This low level of anxiety about the examination process typically occurs among persons who lack motivation for success, are indifferent about a particular career choice, or lack self-discipline. These individuals may have completed a professional program of study but have an insufficient need to succeed as a professional. "If I pass the examination . . . fine . . . but it's not the end of the world if I don't." "It takes too much time and effort to pass the standardized tests; I have better things to do." These hypothetical comments can typify the persons with low anxiety. It is usually only through some major change in life circumstances that instills sufficient anxiety in them to succeed.

However, a much different pattern emerges for persons with high levels of anxiety related to their test performance. Passage of a standardized test is of paramount importance and signifies an end goal for life goals. However, the performance on standardized tests is also low among persons with high levels of anxiety. At this end of the inverted U-shaped curve are persons who often experience debilitating levels of test anxiety. Anxiety itself can diminish cognitive performance and information processing needed to make associations, construct interpretations, and complete operations on information. Highly-anxious individuals often show difficulty in learning material, memory encoding, and retrieval. Test anxiety signals a struggle with a variety of psychological concerns centered on professional progression, fear of failure, fear of success, or long-standing insecurities. The remainder of this chapter is designed to help individuals understand and overcome the negative effects of test anxiety.

Test anxiety is considered to be a specific form of performance anxiety that has multidimensional components (Mueller, 1980). The major components of test anxiety have been identified to be worry and emotionality. Emotionality comprises the sensation of being anxious or nervous accompanied by the physiological signs of anxiety that can include sweating, rapid breathing, blushing, increased heart rate, nausea, headache, gastrointestinal distress, breathing difficulties, frequent urge to urinate, feeling faint, and muscle weakness. These physiological signs are associated with heightened autonomic arousal, both sympathetic and parasympathetic.

Worry signifies the cognitive component of test anxiety and produces a number of impediments to efficiency in the working memory including poor concentration, confused thinking, narrowing of attention, and negative cognitions. Worry produces an acute sensitivity to see danger in many situations regardless if they are objectively dangerous or not. This sensitivity promotes a continual concern about potential harm such as failure on a standardized test and believing passage is beyond the person's capabilities. One failure due to test anxiety may confirm the worries and prevent or impede preparation for reexamination. Reinforcing the worry over potential harm are common negative cognitions that can be seen in statements reflecting on self-doubt and perceived inadequacies that exacerbate a sense of dread or even fear of the testing situation. The negative cognitions can emerge prior to, during, or following the test-taking experience and consequently undermine successful test preparation as well as the completion of the actual examination.

The individuals who experience test anxiety routinely engage in negative self-talk. A common sign of negative self-talk is the repeated use of the phrase "what if." These words emerge in the context of statements that signify self-doubts while adding pressure on the person to succeed. "What if I fail the test? How will I be able to handle my financial debts?" What if I fail the test? Will my family and friends think of me as a loser?" "What if I don't have the time to study for the examination?" What if I become anxious during the examination?"

This "what-if thinking" can begin to dominate the test-anxious individual. It is important to remember that negative self-talk takes place in an automatic fashion and enters one's stream of thought in often subtle ways. As negative self-talk continues it evolves into a telegraphic form. This means that only a single word associated with the "what-if thinking" can come to evoke an entire series of thoughts, past experiences, and memories that heighten anxiety. Self-talk that engenders test anxiety can have an extreme effect on a person as it promotes catastrophic outcomes thinking. The test anxiety-prone person comes to expect failure and expects the worst possible outcomes if failure on the standardized test would occur. The worry aspect of test anxiety can evolve into long-standing characteristics in which the self-talk becomes an automatic process.

Personal Assessment: Identifying the Types of Negative Self-Talk

A categorization of negative self-talkers relevant to the process of test anxiety has been identified by Reid Wilson in his book, *Don't Panic:*

Taking Control of Anxiety Attacks (1996). Recognizing oneself in one of the types can assist in the selection of appropriate intervention strategies for test anxiety.

> The *worrier* is the person who always anticipates the worst, over-estimates the odds that negative outcomes will take place, and imagines the most catastrophic results related to test failure.
> The *critic* is the person with self-talk that is constantly judging and evaluating the individual. Weaknesses or limitations in skills and knowledge are pushed to the mind's forefront at the expense of recognizing positive qualities.
> The *perfectionist* is the person with self-talk that never accepts the current adequacy of knowledge and abilities. No amount of study and preparation is ever enough. This promotes anxiety and feelings that the person "should" always be doing more and more to succeed.

Gaining a good understanding of the underlying process helps in the eventual selection of effective intervention strategies. Although many individuals can accurately articulate their anxiety and the influence it has on their test preparation and taking, not everyone has this clear awareness. People experience test anxiety differently with some persons showing an emphasis on the emotionality component of physical symptoms such as frequent headaches, sleep disturbances, gastrointestinal distress including nausea, and reports of dizziness. Others prominently report worry with an array of cognitive symptoms that can include excessive distractibility, being unable to prioritize study material, misreading of questions, misunderstanding of the questions, focusing away from the test, forgetting basic information, and engaging in negative internal self-talk.

STEP 2: UNDERSTANDING THE MECHANISMS UNDERLYING TEST ANXIETY

Test anxiety has been widely investigated by numerous researchers resulting in an identification of critical factors in this process of worry and emotionality. Understanding the underlying mechanisms that promote and maintain test anxiety can assist in the challenge of overcoming test anxiety and its negative consequences during testing situations. Knowledge and understanding can contribute to the development of a sense of control or personal mastery over such negative states as test anxiety.

Testing as an Aversive Stimulus

"I can't bring myself to buy a study guide."
"I can't even think about the standardized test."
"The thought of the test makes me lose my appetite and have insomnia."

These comments can be common among persons with test anxiety. When the testing situation or anything related to it provokes an uncomfortable or undesirable physiological response, avoidance of the examination has taken place and the responses can be generalized to related stimuli. The experience of test anxiety among many individuals can be explained through the process that the testing situation becomes an aversive stimulus. Persons reacting to the testing situation as an aversive stimulus experience a focus on the emotionality component of test anxiety, as they show a high level of emotional reactivity and heightened arousal states.

The testing situation can become an extremely negative event or an aversive stimulus. Task complexity can reinforce the aversive aspects of the situation. As the importance and difficulty of the test situation increases such as in a standardized test, the aversive qualities are enhanced, which results in heightened emotionality. As with any aversive stimulus, there is then the tendency to avoid the testing situation. Any attempts at studying and preparing for the examination only triggers negative arousal states which in turn interfere with learning. The excessive arousal or anxiety impedes information processing, which exacerbates the negative arousal state. Essentially the test-anxious person becomes overwhelmed by anxiety. The physiological symptom of the emotionality component of anxiety comes to dominate thinking and experience.

Various physiological manifestations of anxiety take over the test-anxious individuals. These symptoms become a detrimental focus of attention, and test-takers that lack appropriate self-regulation abilities cannot effectively cope with uncomfortable physiological responses to the testing situation. Although they may have been successful during lower-stake test situations, the magnitude and importance of a standardized test overwhelms previous coping strategies. Preparation and learning for the test becomes inefficient and inadequate to the point where studying itself can take on aversive qualities leading to the actual avoidance of preparatory activities. This model suggests that for persons with an emphasis on emotionality due to the development of aversion to the testing situation that test anxiety interventions need to adequately address the physiological manifestations.

Skill Deficits and Self-Merit

"I never knew how much I don't know until I began to review for this test."

"I've met students from other programs who seem so prepared for this test."

"I should have spent more time studying when in school instead of having a good time."

Test anxiety can produce a sense of inadequacy in skills and knowledge, which makes a person feel failure on a standardized test is inevitable. For persons falling on the high anxiety end of the inverted U-shaped curve, many believe they possess skills or knowledge deficits. Worry is triggered as a result of the personal assessment that educational and clinical experiences have left the individual ill-prepared for a standardized test. This metacognitive event strikes at the person's sense of competence and questioning of the quality of academic or clinical training. This worry over inadequate preparation produces the worry and negative self-talk that becomes detrimental to the process of achieving success on a standardized test. The test anxiety that results can diminish test performance to the point of failure. Such a negative outcome then serves to prove the underlying worry or questioning of the adequacy of educational and clinical experiences.

Whenever personal assessments lead to worries concerning skill deficits, test anxiety interventions must counteract the negative self-talk related to the worry. Among persons who are qualified for a standardized test, worries about skill deficits are typically due to distortions in thinking caused by anxiety. These individuals benefit from intervention techniques that emphasize productive study habits that reduce anxiety to moderate levels. Cognitive techniques to eliminate negative self-talk should also be used with the improved study skills. With skill enhancement and reduction of negative self-talk, the person is then able to complete an accurate personal assessment of being adequately prepared for standardized test.

"How did I ever think I could become a professional?" This question, which illustrates an auxiliary to the skills deficit issue, is the question of self-merit. As anxiety becomes focused on the examination, some individuals not only question the quality of their academic preparation, but they also become uncertain of their own intellectual capacities. This form of worry serves to attack the person's self-worth and devalues their earlier experiences. Consequently, self-doubt begins to permeate a person's cognitions and the individual develops a sense of being an impostor, or someone who is not worthy to enter a particular profession.

Cognitive Interference

"I can't handle this."
"What if the questions continue to get harder?"
"I can't decide on an answer."
"My mind is a blank . . . what can I do now?"

These are some of the multitude of common comments from persons with test anxiety that can take place *during* an examination. With the presence of test anxiety, the associated worry and emotionality can overwhelm the individual and block concentration and reasoning capacities. Test anxiety increases in its severity as the individual turns away from the actual test questions and toward an internal monologue. When considering testing situations one of the central features differentiating persons who show moderate (beneficial) levels of anxiety on the inverted U-shaped curve to those with high (detrimental) anxiety levels is the presence of cognitive interference and self-depreciative thoughts among the latter. The evaluative nature of a standardized test is a stressor that can produce anxiety. As stated early in the context of the inverted U-shaped curve, moderate anxiety can serve as a motivator and research indicates a high level of achievement among persons at this point on the curve. The high-anxiety test-taker routinely demonstrates poor test performance and often reports test anxiety. According to the cognitive interference approach, the test-taker divides attention between the demands of the testing situation and negative self-talk.

Eventually, the negative thinking overcomes focus on the test demands and negative self-preoccupation takes place.

Among persons with moderate levels of anxiety, the examination is cognitively interpreted as a challenge with anxiety becoming an energizing factor. For the test-anxious individual the test situation is seen as a threat and the anxiety promotes an ever expanding range of negative self-talk. Thus the exact same situation can produce much different outcomes depending upon the amount of anxiety present and how it is handled. The internal monologue or self-talk is a critical factor according to this cognitive interference approach. It is a significant fact that what people say to themselves in their own minds in response to some potentially stressful situation that determines their mood and feelings.

Persons with test anxiety come to believe that the examination situation itself makes them anxious and unable to perform at optimum levels of performance. However, mood is often the result of the thoughts and interpretations each individual makes about a particular event. An important take-away message based on the cognitive interference approach is that each person is largely responsible for how they feel in any given context. Intervention techniques for test anxiety from this perspective will not be effective unless the person accepts the responsibility for their own reactions to potentially stressful events such as a standardized test. The person with test anxiety must accept responsibility and then take charge to practice the techniques and make cognitive modifications in their thinking to gain a sense of mastery over evaluative situations.

Distorted Thinking

Persons with test anxiety due primarily to cognitive interference typically show six basic distortions in their thought processes: overestimation, catastrophic thinking, underestimating coping, overgeneralization, filtering, and emotional reasoning.

The first is an overestimation of negative outcomes. During the examination or while preparing for the test, the person will have intrusive thoughts that emphasize all of the possible negatives to poor test performance.

The second basic distortion is catastrophic thinking, which serves as an extension of overestimation. Catastrophic thinking is an elaboration on the negative outcomes until failure becomes unmanageable and overwhelming. This distortion causes the person with test anxiety to look far beyond the actual testing situation and consider the worst possible long term outcomes. For the test-anxious individual, focusing on the immediacy of the testing situation is lost.

The third distortion is the process of underestimating one's ability to cope. This distortion interacts with catastrophic thinking to promote excessive worry and emotionality to the point when failure on a standardized test becomes inevitable and cannot be undone in future retests. This type of cognitive interference often prevents a person from admitting to test anxiety and seeking help, or it diminishes the likelihood that an intervention strategy will be effective. Thus many individuals may superficially consider remedies for test anxiety but either not follow through on a complete intervention program or half-heartedly pursue a course of action.

The fourth form of distorted thinking is overgeneralization, in which persons with test anxiety come to believe if they had one bad experience, such as failure on an examination due to anxiety, that the failure will come to repeat itself in all future similar situations. The overgeneralization becomes a critical part of cognitive interference through self-talk that consistently uses such words as "never," "always," "everyone," "all," and "nobody." The self-talk takes the form of absolute statements such as, "I'll never be able to pass the examination."

Filtering is the fifth form of distorted thinking that is involved in test anxiety. This distortion becomes apparent when only a single negative aspect of a situation is recognized and the whole is critically evaluated. Filtering produces self-talk that is overloaded with statements that are globally negative and contain such words as "worthless," "pointless," "unjust," "undependable," "incomprehensible," "unproductive," and "valueless." With test anxiety, many useful resources are summarily dismissed through the use of filtering. A series of practice examination questions may be rejected if one is poorly written, or a test intervention technique may be rejected due to one negative comment from another person. The essential problem with test anxiety-generated filtering is that the entirety of a situation is overlooked and poor decision making can result.

The final major form of distorted thinking is termed *emotional reasoning* and refers to the process when situations are evaluated based on emotions and not factual information. This is particularly critical since worry and emotionality are the two key aspects of test anxiety. A person may feel anxious or be experiencing a number of anxiety-related physiological reactions and then base judgments on those sensations. As evaluations are continually made in an emotional fashion, perceptions of the self as being competent diminish. The following statements are common ramifications of emotional reasoning:

"I just feel that I am going to fail on the examination."

"I have to stop using study aids since they make me feel worried."

"I feel so anxious about the examination that I must be an anxious person."

Trait Anxiety

Trait anxiety is often overlooked or ignored as an underlying mechanism involved in test anxiety. Test anxiety is considered to be a state of anxiety that evolves as a learned behavior and is maintained through the mechanisms already discussed above. Many techniques designed to overcome test anxiety focus on the ways to minimize the state of anxiety before, during, and after the testing situation. However, anxiety can also be part of one's personality characteristics, or disposition, and stays with a person regardless of the situation.

Understanding the effects of trait anxiety on those prone to it can also lead to effective interventions to mitigate test anxiety. Trait anxiety is believed to be a relatively stable individual difference in the degree of anxiety proneness. Thus, people display individual differences in their disposition to experience various intensity of anxiety to the same situation or circumstance. Early childhood experiences and innate personality dispositions interact in the development of trait anxiety. With the presence of a dispositional trait toward anxiety, a person has an increased likelihood to show, in a variety of stressful situations, the following signs: *perfectionism, need for approval, need for control, procrastination.*

Perfectionism

With perfectionism, the individual has developed an excessively high level of personal expectations. Seeking to be perfect leads to a pattern of self-defeating thoughts and behaviors. Typically early in life, the person with perfectionism was excessively rewarded for achievement until a personal sense of value could only be obtained when performance was seen as perfect. This striving for perfection leads to a vulnerability and sensitivity to the opinions and criticisms of others. The continual striving for perfection becomes driven through trait anxiety that produces a pattern of negative thinking and beliefs. While trying to attain perfection, the individual's anxiety level is kept at a high level because of thoughts and beliefs dominated by a fear of failure, fear of making mistakes, and a fear of receiving the disapproval of others. Any mistakes are perceived as failures and failure itself diminishes one's sense of personal worth. In addition, if failure takes place the perfectionist believes that rejection and disapproval from other people will follow.

Perfectionism promotes the development of negative self-talk in the form of endless lists of how the person should have done better, or should have done something differently. In this context of fearing failure and fear of not attaining perfect performance, the perfectionist has the daunting task of attempting to attain maximum performance on a standardized test since anything less would signify failure. The trait anxiety brought into the preparation process is then exacerbated through situational aspects of the standardized test that inherently has anxiety-provoking elements. Intervention techniques for perfectionism must focus on challenging the self-defeating negative self-talk it produces and set the stage for the establishment of realistic and attainable goals in the examination process.

Need for Approval

A disposition toward trait anxiety also leads to the presence of an excessive need for approval from other people. A person pursuing recertification or an advanced degree may feel significant pressure for success due to a strong need for approval from family members, a spouse, a partner, or peers. The validation of the individual's self-esteem becomes tied to the passage of a standardized test. Failure to pass the examination would lead to, not only a sense of situational failure, but also to a loss of self-esteem due to the belief that approval from significant others had been lost. Test anxiety develops as both dispositional and situational anxiety cues increase. Need for approval is often associated with the inability to effectively handle critical comments. Learning to accept constructive criticism is the first step in overcoming excessive need for approval and heading off negative self-talk.

Need for Control

Excessive need for control is the desire that everything in life should be predictable. This need is often seen among persons with a high dispositional trait of anxiety. Any situation that may upset the predictability of attaining life goals promotes high levels of anxiety that can be manifest in the form of test anxiety. The requirement to pass a standardized test in order to practice in one's chosen profession adds an element of unpredictability to a person's life goals. Successfully completing professional school comes about following a predictable curriculum and clinical experiences. However, that predictable path toward professional practice can be derailed through failure on an examination. Failure on an exam can lead to serious questions about future professional practice taking place within an acceptable timeframe or even at all.

With the existence of excessive need for control comes a sense of vulnerability around anxiety-provoking situations such as an examination. That vulnerability enhances the experience of anxiety together with the worry and emotionality associated with test anxiety. It should be noted that persons with excessive need for control are particularly vulnerable to experiencing a drastic reaction to failure on an examination. Failure could send the person into a sense of chaos in which life goes out of control. For persons with excessive need for control it is important to manage this manifestation of trait anxiety in order to avoid the detrimental effects of failure. Intervention needed to overcome excessive need for control must be practiced for the long term and involve establishing cognitions that emphasize patience, acceptance of reality as it comes, and trust in one's capabilities.

Procrastination

The avoidance of a particular task that needs to be completed is termed procrastination. Many people have the tendency toward procrastination and the causes are many. If a task is seen as lacking personal relevance, there is a tendency to postpone its completion. When the nature of the task is ambiguous or has been imposed upon a person unfairly, procrastination is a common response. However, procrastination can emerge for highly-structured relevant tasks that are directly related to a person's life goals. This is true when a person must pass a standardized examination. Many individuals with a high dispositional anxiety trait become particularly uncomfortable in situations with an evaluative component such as an examination. In an attempt to diminish the trait anxiety, individuals may try to ignore the test, underestimate the work needed to prepare adequately for the examination, find distractions to be removed from tasks associated with the test, or minimize the difficulty of the examination. Interventions to overcome procrastination are designed around developing an effective time management strategy that clearly establishes steps toward the goal and ways to monitor progress effectively.

STEP 3: OVERCOMING TEST ANXIETY THROUGH INTERVENTIONS

Three phases in the learning–testing cycle have been identified and test anxiety interventions are appropriate in each. Test preparation, test performance, and test reflection comprise the three phases. High levels of test anxiety have a detrimental effect on a person in all three phases of the cycle. The worry and emotionality associated with test anxiety maintained in each phase impacts negatively on examination outcomes. Understanding the learning–testing cycle can assist in the implementation of appropriate interventions for test anxiety.

Test Preparation

During the test preparation phase, individuals with test anxiety experience problems in effectively encoding material that needs to be learned for the examination. This produces insufficient cognitive processing that would permit achieving an effective conceptual understanding of the subject matter. Teaching a learner an effective study strategy to assist with encoding of material and its storage can overcome any skills deficit in this arena, but it does not completely alleviate the deleterious effects of test anxiety. The many other underlying mechanisms of test anxiety continue to negatively impact on the learner.

Test Performance

The traditional focus on handling test anxiety has been in this phase of the learning–testing cycle. Strategies to assist a test-taker have focused on interventions designed to overcome task interference, but this overlooks the connection between the phases in the learning–testing cycle. The most effective interventions for test anxiety are multidimensional across the cycle.

Test Reflection

Each learner experiences a period of reflection on the testing situation. This may take place following experience with the actual examination, one of its practice tests, or a debriefing session with someone who also took the test. It is at this point that the learner experiences the worry and emotionality associated with test anxiety. This maintains both the cognitions and physiological reactions that have been discussed previously and supports the notion that intervention strategies need to be practiced throughout the learning–testing cycle.

General Interventions in the Learning–Testing Cycle

In the context of the learning–testing cycle, there has been a long tradition of standard recommendations to reduce test anxiety. In the test preparation phase, a person is advised to increase self-confidence through a study program that is paced and comprehensive with material broken into meaningful segments to be covered at specific intervals of time. Progress in learning the material needs to be continually assessed through the posing of questions as each segment of material is reviewed. Cramming is considered to be an ineffective form of studying and must be avoided in the test preparation phase. Studying is optimal when a moderate pace is maintained that permits breaks and continuance of recreational and social activities.

Throughout the test preparation phase, healthy habits of good nutrition and exercise need to be maintained as well as good sleep and hygiene. Avoid excessive use of any substances that may compromise encoding and consolidation of study material or distract from the study process. To help modify anxiety, avoidance of anxious peers who also may be planning to take the examination should take place. The use of study groups or a study partner can have a number of benefits to assist in the monitoring progress of mastering the material but only if the others involved do not foster anxiety or negative self-talk.

Examination day needs to be preceded by a restful evening and greeted with a nutritious breakfast. Allow for a leisurely commute to the testing location and a period of relaxation to calm the mind immediately prior to the examination. Avoid any contacts with other people or situations that may trigger anxiety or negative self-talk. Focus thoughts on assuring yourself that test preparation has been accomplished successfully. At the time of testing, monitoring one's internal state can be accomplished to ensure that cognitive interference is not impeding test performance. Be prepared to talk to yourself during the examination with scripted comments that prevent or control negative self-talk. The goal is to remain focused on the examination questions rather than on worry and emotionality.

The test reflection phase can be a critical period that could significantly affect subsequent testing. Focus on making an objective assessment of the study plan that was followed. Identify what went well and what could be improved upon. Consider the effectiveness of the methods that were used to control worry and emotionality. Make a commitment to formulate an individualized intervention plan for exam preparation and control of test anxiety if a reexamination is to take place. Stop any tendencies toward catastrophic thinking. Instead, reward yourself for completing an objective test reflection.

The remainder of this chapter focuses on appropriate intervention techniques that can be combined to establish a multidimensional strategy to counteract the underlying mechanisms of test anxiety and overcome the worry and emotionality associated with it. Read the subsequent sections with the goal of identifying the major test-anxiety issues impacting on your personal testing experiences. Remember that intervention strategies for test anxiety are most effective when a combination is utilized that addresses the underlying mechanisms predominant in one's personal makeup.

TESTING AS AN AVERSIVE STIMULUS: INTERVENTIONS

As discussed previously, the emotionality component of test anxiety involves a wide array of physiological reactions that can overwhelm an individual's normal coping capacities prior to and during the examination situation. As a means to gain control of these physical manifestations of anxiety, *progressive muscle relaxation* can be very effective. Progressive relaxation targets the muscle tension that is one physical reaction to anxiety. If a person can experience a relaxation of the muscle tension, the associated feelings of anxiety diminish. It must be remembered that the positive outcomes of this technique are obtained in a gradual fashion. For a person to gain a sense of mastery using this technique, it must be practiced consistently. Calming music can serve as a useful adjunct to the process of achieving progressive muscle relaxation. Reaping the benefits of progressive muscle relaxation requires a daily routine that takes place at a regular time of at least 20 minutes twice daily. A quiet location is needed that is free of unusual distractions. A comfortable position and loose attire should be the norm as the mind is freed of worry and tension. A series of exercises are employed involving the contracting and relaxing of various muscle groups across the entire body. There are a number of progressive muscle relaxation sequences available to follow toward total body relaxation. A primary source for progressive muscle relaxation can be found in *The Relaxation and Stress Reduction Workbook* (Davis, Eshelman, & McKay, 2000).

Abdominal breathing is often considered to be a foundation for progressive muscle relaxation. Shallow breathing that is rapid and high in the chest is often a sign of tension. A relaxed form of breathing takes place fully, deeply from the abdomen. It is difficult to maintain an anxious tense state when practicing abdominal breathing thus it can help trigger a relaxation response. At the first indications of the emotionality associated with test anxiety, engaging abdominal breathing can be the first step in averting an escalation of symptoms. Calming breathing exercises can be found in a classic book, *Beyond the Relaxation Response* (Benson & Proctor, 1985).

In combination with progressive relaxation, *visualization* is often used to reduce anxiety. Visualization involves forming mental images that promote relaxation, or are imagined scenes of success. Visualization is an ability to produce mental pictures in one's mind that are vivid and realistic. The mental image promotes a positive change in a person's emotionality. Practicing visualization can increase the vividness of the images and the ease at which an image can be attained. Visualization has even been used successfully to help professional practice clinical procedures. It is also a well-known technique used among athletes to maximize performance. Athletes routinely gain a sense of mastery over the action to be performed through visualizing successful outcomes.

Forming images that are restful, like walking along a secluded beach, can facilitate the attainment of a relaxed state. The use of visualization can establish an ideal sense of calm and relaxation that coincides with a specific imagined image. Because people with test anxiety exhibit emotionality, putting yourself in a calming imagined scene blocks the physiological manifestations of test anxiety. The underlying assumption is that a state of relaxation is an incompatible response to anxiety. Imagining yourself as being calm and relaxed in the testing situation can serve to overcome the emotionality usually experienced in such a circumstance. Practicing relaxation with a specific imagined scene allows the use of that particular image as a cue for attaining calmness in times of stress. A number of visualization and guided imagery scenarios can be found in the book, *Visualization for Change* (Fanning, 1994).

SKILLS DEFICIT AND SELF-MERIT: INTERVENTIONS

Anyone who uses this book has already identified the importance of learning specific skills related to successful test-taking. Learning to orient yourself to the particular demands of a specific standardized test has been addressed previously in this book. Understanding the purposes of a specific test, the construction of the test questions, using practice examination questions, and good study habits all fit together to promote optimal examination performance. Success comes from learning to think about one's own thinking (metacognition) while knowing how to counteract the detrimental influences of worry and emotionality coming from test anxiety. Metacognition is optimal when test anxiety has been controlled and is out of the high end of the inverted U-shaped curve discussed previously.

Cueing can keep a test-taker from becoming overwhelmed with test anxiety when encountering difficult questions. This technique involves analyzing examination questions and answer options to identify the information the learner actually knows about the content involved. A general principle is that a difficult question often promotes test anxiety; therefore, it becomes aversive and is not examined closely. However, carefully reviewing the content of difficult questions, through well-placed guiding questions, typically elicits recognition that the learner is more knowledgeable about the material than previously believed. Carefully analyzing practice questions to display knowledge and understanding of the various parts demonstrates the importance of taking an approach of critically reviewing examination questions seen as difficult or impossible to answer. Such questions should be broken down into parts so that the learner can identify content they do know and garner a sense of mastery of the content. This process helps to overcome the emotionality and worry that often can emerge from self-doubts and thoughts that diminish self-merit (Veenman, Keseboom, & Imthorn, 2000).

Even though an individual may have used successful strategies for testing situations in the past, the magnitude of the importance of passing a standardized test can lead to self-doubts and worry. To counteract the intrusions of self-doubt and negative self-talk, many individuals who are prone to test anxiety benefit from revisiting some classic examples of effective study habits. Following a specific study system during the test preparation phase of the learning–testing cycle can help to minimize emotionality and the cognitive interference of negative self-talk. Utilizing study systems can help to build a confidence in one's knowledge while facilitating the encoding and storage of examination related content.

The following are two study systems that have a significant body of research supporting their effectiveness. Readers are advised to seek the specifics about study systems using the references provided for each.

The ASPIRE Study System was developed by Dwayne Ross, Edward R. Wilkens, and Phyllis Utley. The components of this approach are as follows: A: approach, attitude, arrange; S: select, survey, study; P: put aside, piece together; I: inspect, investigate, inquire; R: reconsider reflect, relay; E: evaluate, examine, explore. The ASPIRE study system provides a good framework to organize the material to be reviewed during the test preparation phase of the learning–testing cycle and is available at the study guide's website: www.studygs.net.

The MURDER Study System is similar to ASPIRE but has fewer steps due to a condensation of some of the points found in the latter approach. The MURDER system guides the learner through the following steps: M: mood (positive); U: understanding; R: recall (putting in own words); D: digest (and reconsideration); E: expand (through questioning); and R. review. The specifics of this study system can be obtained in the book, *The Complete Problem Solver* (Hayes, 1989).

COGNITIVE INTERFERENCE: INTERVENTIONS

People who experience test anxiety usually show problems with working memory during the examination situation. When anxiety reaches the high end of the inverted U-shaped curve, the individual will have a difficult time retrieving the content that was studied. This experience produces such statements as, "I knew the material but my mind just went blank." During the test reflection phase, it is typical for the person to then regain full memory of the information. This phenomenon triggers negative self-talk and reinforces the worry component of test anxiety. It should noted that this "blanking" can also be seen during the test preparation phase when excessive anxiety can be triggered by difficult study content or emergence of negative self-talk. The result of experiencing test anxiety in the test preparation phase is that it diminishes the knowledge base and sets the stage for high levels of worry during the test performance phase. The person with test anxiety experiences interference with storage and processing of the examination content.

To overcome these negative effects, it is useful to use strategies that assist information processing and memory. Using mnemonics is a traditional method to improve organization and recall of exam content. Games have also been used to assist in the test preparation phase. Many study guides present examination relevant information in the form of crossword puzzles or *Jeopardy!*-style question and answer formats. Such games would not be the focus of preparation for the examination, but they could serve the function of diminishing anxiety before it reaches a point of inhibiting test preparation. If a person is experiencing information and memory processing difficulties, it is useful to learn to ask questions using practice questions. This metacognitive process of cueing was discussed in a previous chapter.

The self-talk that intrudes into the conscious mind takes a person away from the examination questions into a pattern of negative thinking. A variety of cognitive techniques have been identified that help to overcome the self-talk that is related to test anxiety. *Cognitive restructuring* is the process of challenging irrational negative thinking and replacing it with realistic thoughts. This process involves the following steps.

- Record
- Review
- Challenge
- Problem solve
- Restructure

Record. It is important for the individual with test anxiety to identify the negative thoughts that interfere with intellectual performance. In this technique, a log or diary listing and describing the negative thoughts is created. Guiding statements in writing the log are, "Whenever I feel anxious about the board examination, I begin thinking about. . . ." "The idea of preparing for the board examination makes me think about. . . ." "The thought of sitting down to take the board examination makes me think or feel. . . ."

Review. The comments written in the log are made concrete with the possibility of reviewing them for completeness and details. This provides the initial opportunity to evaluate the potentially intrusive self-talk that emerges among persons with test anxiety who will begin to gain a sense of control over their thoughts.

Challenge. The content of the negative self-talk can now be challenged through such questions as "What actual evidence exists that the negative outcome will take place?" "Do I have to freeze when confronted with difficult examination questions?" "Are self-doubts so powerful they can stop me from succeeding?" "Haven't I learned to solve other problems in my life?" "I don't have to be controlled by what other people think of me."

Problem Solve. After challenging the negative cognitions, a focus toward finding solutions can take place. Attacking symptoms, such as catastrophic thinking, that emerge during negative self-talk, with real solutions, can diminish anxiety. "There are specifics I can do to refocus during the examination rather than freeze; I will use the technique of. . . ." "I can learn to remain relaxed and focused by learning to. . . ."

Restructure. Once again, it is important to recall that moderate levels of anxiety are beneficial for maximum performance on examinations. It is not necessary, nor is it desirable, to completely eliminate anxiety prior to taking a standardized test. What is important is to feel in sufficient control of anxiety so that when it emerges the feelings can be utilized as a motivator toward achievement rather than failure. After problem solving, the worry about test anxiety can be restructured to a sense of control with the confidence of having a repertoire of techniques to avert the negatives of test anxiety: "It's helpful and tells me to spend additional time on a specific content area." "Feeling some anxiety is normal and I can use it to my benefit." "Anxiety doesn't need to be inhibiting, it can be energizing." Specific details about the cognitive restructuring process can be found in an excellent resource book, *Taking the Anxiety Out of Taking Tests* (Johnson, 2000).

DISTORTED THINKING: INTERVENTIONS

As described earlier in this chapter, distorted thinking can interfere with test preparation and test performance in the form of overestimation of a negative outcome, catastrophic thinking, underestimation of coping capacity, overgeneralization that negative outcomes will repeat, cognitive filtering of positives with focus on negatives, and emotional reasoning.

Test anxiety promotes negative self-talk that significantly interferes with test preparation and test performance, as well as poisons the test reflection phase. Not all negative self-talk is the same for all people with test anxiety. The nature of personal worry and individual life circumstances can influence the content of the negative self-talk and the form of the cognitive distortion that occurs. Although content may differ, the negative thinking is always detrimental to the desired outcome of passing a standardized test. In order to effectively handle the negative self-talk, *counterstatements* to the cognitive distortions must be developed. Positive and supportive statements that are counter to the self-talk serve as interventions to the cognitive interference produced by cognitive distortions.

The *counterstatement technique* involves writing down and then rehearsing positive statements that directly dismiss or discredit negative self-talk. It is important to monitor self-talk to identify examples of filtering and other cognitive distortions. Recognition of the content permits the development of rational counterstatements. Creating charts listing the specific negative self-talk statements that emerge when test anxiety worry emerges is necessary so that a positive counterstatement can be entered on the chart alongside each negative statement. When reviewing the negative self-statements due to distortions, pay particular attention to those with an emphasis on "should." "I should get all the questions correct." "I should never be worried." Worry and emotionality feed upon "should" statements. Be realistic in developing counterstatements to the "should" comments. In general, the development of counterstatements involves the process of challenging the underlying foundations of negative thinking. Common challenges to negative statements would be, "What is the evidence? Is this always true? Am I looking at the whole picture? Am I being objective?"

Be prepared with counterstatements so that when worry and emotionality are initially perceived, the negative cognitive distortions can be pushed aside. When experiencing test anxiety, negative self-statements usually have a strong hold on an individual, thus it is important to practice counterstatements often and keep them in the present tense with strong "I" statements attached. "I can learn all of the material." "I know how to study effectively." "I am willing to do whatever it takes to succeed." Detailed instructions on using specific procedures to develop counterstatements can be found in the resource book, *The Self-Talk Solution* (Helmstetter, 1990).

TRAIT ANXIETY: INTERVENTIONS

As noted earlier in this chapter, some individuals have a disposition toward experiencing higher levels of anxiety than other people in the same situations. This dispositional trait of anxiety can lead to factors that inhibit attaining maximum test performance including: perfectionism, excessive need for approval, need for control, and procrastination.

These conditions serve to exacerbate the worry and emotionality of test anxiety. A number of techniques can be used to help control dispositional trait anxiety.

For the person with *perfectionistic* tendencies, it is beneficial for the individual to shift focus away from ideas that reinforce the notion that only perfect performance is permissible. The perfectionist usually believes that personal worth is only gained through achievements and overlooks the inherent value of a human being. The perfectionist must challenge the belief system, which dictate that it is only through exceptional achievements that a person gains value in the eyes of others.

The person showing perfectionism also overreacts to small mistakes and focuses on small insufficiencies. An effective way to handle this aspect of perfectionism is to direct attention to accomplishments, both large and small. Successes can be attained without perfect performance and the outcomes can be identical. Practicing to change one's cognitions about what constitutes success and setting realistic goals are needed to diminish the potentially anxiety provoking aspects of perfectionism.

Excessive *need for approval* from others often promotes apprehension and worry. To overcome the need to be approved by others, the anxious person needs to recognize the codependency that exists and learn to break free of the bonds. The excessive need for approval can be indicated through such statements as: "I must keep people I love happy." "I need to do whatever it takes to keep this relationship." "I should not do anything to make someone angry at me." These types of statements, which become part of a person's self-talk, serve to keep anxiety high and stimulate a need to remain vigilant against doing anything that could produce disapproval. To intervene against the excessive need for approval, a person needs to effectively challenge the underlying beliefs and take care of oneself. Codependency has to be rejected in favor of such self-care statements as: "I can accept the way I am." "I don't need to worry about what others want me to do." "I have my own needs."

The underlying motivation for *need for control* of one's surroundings is a need for order and predictability in life. If life is without surprises, then limited stress associated with the unknown should be experienced. However, an excessive need for control typically signals an underlying disposition of anxiety as a person strives to minimize life stressors. Testing or evaluative situations bring about worry and emotionality.

Once experiencing an excessive need for control, a person responds by seeking as much order in life as possible. Unfortunately, as the uncertainties of the testing situation draw near, the worry and emotionality of test anxiety grow with the concern that examination outcome cannot be adequately controlled. Cognitive interference emerges as self-doubt grows in the person coinciding with the worry and emotionality of test anxiety.

Interventions for excessive need for control revolve around accepting the uncertainties of life and developing patience. The interventions are cognitively-based with a combined focus on relaxation techniques to control emotionality and challenging the need for control. The goal is to achieve a cognitive state that would endorse statements such as, "I am comfortable with life's uncertainties."

Procrastination is often a sign of a disposition toward anxiety. Fear of what lies ahead can trigger the many delaying behaviors associated with procrastination. The time-honored interventions to combat procrastination include developing effective time management skills that provide an orderly plan for test preparation and strategies for the test performance phase (see Chapter 6 for additional information).

In summary, realizing that trait anxiety can serve as foundation for situational test anxiety is an important first step in selecting the tools to keep this component in check. Make an honest assessment for the presence of a dispositional component to test anxiety, and then accept the challenge to modify the long-standing personal assumptions that produced and maintain the anxiety trait. Understand that if specific anxiety reduction techniques are ineffective, individual counseling may be a beneficial step to consider (McKay, Davis, & Fanning, 1998).

SUMMARY

As has been discussed, test anxiety has the capacity to produce failure among people taking a standardized test through the process of worry and emotionality. Test anxiety produces restrictions in working memory capacity to a degree that it significantly diminishes cognitive performance during the test preparation, test performance, and test reflection phases. Self-talk that is task irrelevant and negative thinking occupy the working memory and prevent adequate information processing. The purpose of this chapter was to make you aware of the signs and symptoms of test anxiety, explain the underlying mechanisms of test anxiety, and direct you to appropriate interventions to overcome the detrimental effects of anxiety. The good news about test anxiety is that it can be effectively overcome making success on a standardized test within reach.

SECTION IV SUMMARY AND NEXT STEPS

In Section IV—*Executing Your Game Plan*—we recommended methods and techniques to help you achieve the highest score that you can; the score that you deserve after all your hard work!

Before proceeding with the rest of this book, please reflect on the following questions:

- What was the primary take-away message for you from this chapter?
- What information will be the easiest for you to include in your exam preparation?

Be sure to complete the Chapter 12 Activity before starting to read the Epilogue.

CHAPTER 12 ACTIVITY

Working With and Through Test Anxiety

Chapter 12—*Managing Test Anxiety*—discussed the detrimental effects that test anxiety can have on test scores and presented interventions to minimize its impact. Effective concentration is an important factor in one's preparation for a high stakes standardized examination and can ultimately help reduce test anxiety. Assess your concentration level using the following template, and then devise ways to improve it.

Table	
12–1	**Activity 1**

a. How often does your attention wander away from the study topic at hand?

b. How often to you think about the outcome of your test rather than your preparation?

c. When you depart from a task do you return to complete it?

d. When you choose a strategic goal, do you persist in your efforts until you achieve it?

e. Do your tactical changes involve adding to or subtracting from your study plan?

f. Do you spend a lot of time worrying rather than doing?

Epilogue: Executive Summary of Book

Knowing is not the same thing as doing. You can know there are study techniques that will help you score higher on an examination. You can know about techniques that enhance your ability to memorize and recall information. You can know that some study techniques are more effective than others. You can know that self-regulating individuals tend to be higher performers on standardized tests. You can know all of these things and much more. It's not what you know that matters most; it's what you do with your knowledge that makes the difference.

There's a lot of information in this book. There's a lot more information in the literature that we cited and even more in the literature that we could not include in our book. In closing, we selected 12 topics that were described in this book and ranked them from #1—the most likely to increase your test score, to #12—fundamentally important, but not enough. Please review the list and quiz yourself as follows:

- Do I know what this term or phrase means?
- Do I plan to incorporate this concept into my study plan?
- Do I plan to practice and refine this skill?
- Who can I talk with to learn more about the items from this list that I choose to pursue?
  #1—Self-Regulation
  #2—Group Studying with a PAL
  #3—Improved Self Efficacy

#4—Moderated Test Anxiety
#5—Focused and Timely Feedback
#6—Time Management
#7—Goals and Objectives
#8—Test-Wiseness
#9—Test-Taking Skills
#10—Diversified Study Behaviors
#11—Self-created Study Aids
#12—Memorization of Content/Rehearsal Studying Techniques

We hope that you know a lot more about standardized tests and how to study for them after reading our book. We are passionate about what we do and are optimistic that our experiences, suggestions, and recommendations will help you as you prepare for your upcoming standardized test(s). Now that you know about what to do, please complete Exercise 3 so that you can plan what *you will do*. Exercises 1 and 2 may be found in the Roadmap of this book.

Best wishes as you prepare for your upcoming standardized test.

EXERCISE 3

Finalizing Your Study Plan

It's time to finalize your study plan. Review the comments you wrote in Exercise 1—*Drafting Your Study Plan*—when you started reading this book. We hope that your answers are now much more explicit and robust than they were the first time. This document will constitute your final study plan. Follow it. Modify it. ***Good luck***.

EXERCISE 3A

Some Guidance for Your Final Study Plan

If you need assistance completing your study plan, here are the chapters in which you will find information that can help you individualize your approach (see Table EM-2).

Table	
EM–1	Exercise 3

Questions

1. What study techniques will I use to prepare for this test?

2. Which books, computer programs, study aids, and the like will I use to help me prepare?

3. How much total time will I study for this test; how long will I study each day?

4. When will I start studying for this test?

5. What can I do on the day of the test to increase my score?

6. As the test approaches, how will I know that I am almost ready?

Table	
EM–2	Exercise 3A

Questions

1. What study techniques will I use to prepare for this test?
   Refer to Chapters 1, 2, 5, 7, 8, and 9.

2. Which books, computer programs, study aids, and the like, will I use to help me prepare?
   Refer to Chapters 2, 3, 5, and 9.

3. How much total time will I study for this test; how long will I study each day?
   Refer to Chapters 2 and 5.

4. When will I start studying for this test?
   Refer to Chapters 1, 6, and 8.

5. What can I do on the day of the test to increase my score?
   Refer to Chapters 10, 11, and 12.

6. As the test approaches, how will I know that I am getting ready?
   Refer to Chapters 4, 6, 8, and 9.

Appendix

A

Standardized Test Websites

The following list of standardized test websites should prove useful to you.

ACT (American College Testing)
Home page: http://www.act.org/
Facts about ACT: http://www.act.org/news/ aapfacts.html

COMLEX (Comprehensive Osteopathic Medical Licensing Examination)
Home page: http://nbome.org/
Facts about COMLEX: http://nbome.org/docs/ comlexBOI.pdf

DAT (Dental Admission Test)
Home page: http://www.ada.org/dat.aspx
Facts about DAT: http://www.ada.org/sections/ educationAndCareers/pdfs/info_dat_practice_ test.pdf

GED (General Educational Development)
Home page: http://www.acenet.edu/AM/ Template.cfm?Section=GED_TS
Facts about GED: http://www.acenet.edu/ Content/NavigationMenu/ged/faq/index.htm

EPPP (Examination for Professional Practice of Psychology)
Home page: http://www.asppb.net/i4a/pages/ index.cfm?pageid=3279
Facts about the EPPP: http://www.asppb.net/i4a/ pages/index.cfm?pageid=3433

GMAT (Graduate Management Admission Test)
Home page: http://www.mba.com
Facts about GMAT: http://www.gmac.com/gmac/thegmat/gmatbasics/

GRE (Graduate Records Examination)
Home page: http://www.ets.org/gre/
Facts about GRE: http://www.ets.org/gre/revised_general/faq/

LSAT (Law School Admission Council)
Home page: http://www.lsac.org/
Facts about LSAT: http://www.lsac.org/JD/LSAT/about-the-LSAT.asp

MCAT (Medical College Admission Test)
Home page: https://www.aamc.org/students/applying/mcat/
Facts about MCAT: https://www.aamc.org/students/applying/mcat/about/

NAPLEX (North American Pharmacist Licensure Examination)
Home page: http://www.nabp.net/programs/examination/naplex/index.php
Facts about NAPLEX: http://www.nabp.net/programs/examination/naplex/naplex-faqs/

NCLEX (National Council Licensure Examination)
Home page: https://www.ncsbn.org/nclex.htm
Facts about NCLEX: https://www.ncsbn.org/2321.htm

PANCE (Physician Assistant National Certifying Examination)
Home page: http://www.nccpa.net/Pance.aspx
Facts about PANCE: http://www.nccpa.net/faq.aspx#1

PANRE (Physician Assistant National Recertifying Examination)
Home page: http://www.nccpa.net/Panre.aspx
Facts about PANRE: http://www.nccpa.net/faq.aspx#5

PCAT (Pharmacy College Admission Test)
Home page: http://www.pearsonassessments.com/haiweb/Cultures/en-US/site/Community/PostSecondary/Products/pcat/pcathome.htm
Facts about PCAT: http://www.pearsonassessments.com/hai/Images/dotCom/pcatweb.info/PCAT_CBT_FAQ2011.pdf

SAT (Scholastic Aptitude Test or Scholastic Assessment Test)
Home page: http://www.collegeboard.org/

Facts about SAT: http://www.collegeboard.com/prod_downloads/sat/sat-facts.pdf

USMLE (United States Medical Licensing Examination)
Home page: http://www.usmle.org/
Facts about USMLE: http://www.usmle.org/General_Information/FAQs/FAQs-General.html

Appendix

B
Essay Questions: A Game Plan

We encourage you to review the website of the standardized test you will be taking to familiarize yourself with the parameters of the exam. In order to be prepared, you need to know if the test will include an essay component. In addition, be aware of the methodology that will be used to score your essay (see Appendix A: *Standardized Test Websites*).

Essay questions provide insight into your ability to (1) understand and interpret directions (i.e., do what the question asks), (2) recall relevant information (e.g., remember facts and concepts), (3) reason (i.e., create an original and meaningful answer using higher-order thinking), and (4) effectively communicate your thought processes in writing (i.e., compose an organized and clear response using proper grammar, punctuation, and appropriate vocabulary). The good news is that most of the same test preparation principles and practices described throughout this book can also prepare you to write a high-scoring essay on test day.

If the exam you will be taking has a writing (essay) component, do not disregard its importance. When standardized test scores are evaluated as part of an admission application process, a strong performance on the multiple-choice (objective) portion of an exam may only place you into a pool of equally qualified applicants. The writing component of the standardized examination is often used to help admission personnel differentiate among the individuals within a pool of qualified applicants (Hill, Hynes, Joyce, & Green, 2011). In other words, it has the potential to set you apart from the rest. Before describing some specific writing strategies to use on exam day, let's first consider some fundamental information about essay examinations.

THE BASICS

The essential element of an essay question is that it requires you to *compose your response* to a posed question or problem, rather than simply select an answer from among a group of options. Furthermore, in contrast to multiple-choice questions (MCQs), there is no single best answer. Essay questions more readily (than MCQs) assess cognitive flexibility and higher-order thinking skills, such as the ability to analyze, apply, compare, infer, interpret, predict, defend, develop, evaluate, explain, justify, and propose. An examinee that has prepared well—in other words, used study techniques that foster deep learning, understanding, and long-term retention—should be able to demonstrate efficiency with these skills when reasoning through an essay question.

Essays are usually seen by examinees as difficult due to the need to write an original, well-organized response within a limited amount of time. This can be a daunting task even for practiced writers. Essay questions on standardized examinations allow for a variety of different response patterns and typically permit examinees to structure their answers with very few guidelines. Therefore, developing a game plan before exam day will help take some of the pressure off, allowing you to use your exam time more efficiently. In fact, understanding how to structure an essay can allow you to write a reasonable response even on a subject with which you are not particularly familiar.

Critical Thinking and Essay Type

When you come face-to-face with an essay question, read it carefully and make sure you *follow the directions* (Reiner, Bothell, Sudweeks, & Wood, 2002). Failure to accomplish this rudimentary task is a primary, and easily preventable, reason for poor performance on essay examinations. In addition to providing direction for organizing your response, Davis (2009) describes that certain words provide *clues to the critical thinking skills* you need to display in your answer. Moss & Holder (1988) refer to these words as "directive verbs" and they include words such as analyze, compare, evaluate, interpret, justify, prove, or summarize. Make sure you know what each of these different directive verbs mean. If you don't, part of your preparation process should include looking them up in a dictionary. These words help provide context to your response—they give you your task, the job you need to accomplish—and they should guide your thought process as you frame your answer. Recognizing the type of essay question you are being asked to write is an important first step in producing an effective response. There are four basic types of essays: factual, analysis, synthesis, and opinion.

Factual essay questions require the examinee to demonstrate recall and understanding of factual knowledge. The directions may ask the examinee to state, trace, describe, or summarize.

Analysis essay questions go beyond presentation of factual information and require the examinee to explain or discuss relationships such as cause and effect. Directive verbs include words such as analyze, evaluate, explain, compare/contrast, or discuss.

Synthesis essay questions assess the higher-order reasoning skills that enable the examinee to apply or transfer knowledge learned in one context to a different context. The directions could include such words as relate, illustrate, prove, justify, or interpret.

The *opinion essay* is the only type of essay in which it is appropriate to express your opinion. Typically you would be asked to take a position on a specific topic or controversial issue. Although the opinion essay permits greater freedom in expressing one's own point of view, the examinee should still make every effort to demonstrate critical thinking skills. The development of your response should answer a question such as "What evidence, observations, or experiences led you to and provide support for your opinion?"

Planning and Completing Your Response

Once the directions have been read at least twice and the type of essay question has been determined, it is time to formulate your response. A basic essay has three sections: introduction, middle (body), and conclusion. The introduction is where you state the central idea of the essay, otherwise known as the *thesis*. The middle section or body of the essay *provides explanation and support for the central idea*. This is the longest part of the essay and requires organization as well as critical thinking and reasoning skills. Most of the knowledge-based information (e.g., facts, details, concepts) is provided in this section. The conclusion is where you summarize your arguments and evidence for the central idea and make your closing comments. Structurally, the conclusion should tie closely to the introduction as it brings the central idea, first stated in the introduction, to its logically derived summation.

Although some examinees believe it is a waste of time to plan their response before beginning, we contend that planning can make the difference between a well-organized, thoughtful answer and a rambling, pointless one.

Be mindful of the time allotted for you to complete the essay question and take just a few moments to consider your approach and construct a brief outline. In order to achieve a high score on an essay question, your response must express specific, relevant knowledge in a manner that demonstrates your higher-order critical thinking skills. It cannot simply be a series of facts strung together. Even a factual essay should be organized and present a logical flow of information. Preparing an outline to guide your thinking and writing will help you create an organized and logical essay. Think of the outline as a game plan that will help you strategize for the completion of the best possible essay, or as a road map that can keep you from getting lost.

There are two types of outlines you might find helpful: topic outlines and graphic outlines. It doesn't matter which type you choose, but we strongly recommend you select one. Outlines provide a skeleton or overview of your planned response and serve as a template to help you remember where to address the important elements of your essay. Topic outlines are a standard form of outline with which most people are familiar, consisting of major and minor headings and subheadings organized in a hierarchical fashion (see Figure EM-1). Graphic outlines (similar to concept maps; refer to Chapter 9 to review concept maps) are a more visual representation of the relationships between pieces of information (see Figure EM-2 for an example on reducing the risk of a heart attack). If you are a strong visual learner, consider drawing a simple diagram to complement your outline and serve as a visual cue to help you focus on the central point and its development toward a logical conclusion.

Figure EM-1

Topic Outline (Template)

1. Introduction
   a. Restate the question posed in an engaging first sentence that captures your reader's interest
   b. State the central idea or thesis of your essay (e.g., your answer to the question in general terms)
   c. Write a sentence that describes how you will address the question
2. Body
   a. Point 1
      i. Explanation 1
      ii. Supporting example 1
   b. Point 2
      i. Explanation 2
      ii. Supporting example 2 (as needed)
   c. Point 3
      i. Explanation 3
      ii. Supporting example 3 (as needed)
3. Conclusion
   a. Summarize your response by tying the preceding facts and thoughts together
   b. End with a powerful and convincing final comment

Once a very basic outline has been completed, think of examples or specific details that will support the central idea of the essay. Make a notation in your outline where the examples will best fit in order to demonstrate logical sequencing of ideas and critical thinking skills. As you write you will flesh out the skeleton by adding details to your outline. To enhance the effectiveness of your outline, it can be helpful to place some directive verbs at different points to remind you of the critical thinking skills you will be expected to demonstrate (e.g., analyze, compare and contrast, justify, and prove) based on the type of essay you are expected to compose.

The introduction of your essay should be designed to "catch the attention" of an impartial reader. The first sentence or two should indicate to the reader that you understand the question and are proceeding

Figure EM-2

Graphic Outline: Reducing the Risk of a Heart Attack

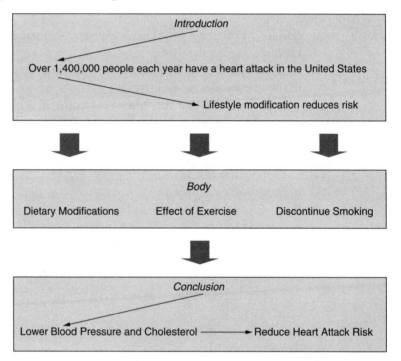

with a relevant point or argument. If you are having trouble getting started, simply begin by rephrasing the question as a statement. It is important to use clear, unambiguous language. Your thesis (central idea) must both satisfy the directions for the essay and be obvious to a reader. Remember that no matter how effectively you state your central point or thesis, if it does not address the task laid out in the question, it will likely receive a low score. If you're really having a hard time beginning, it may be useful to write your conclusion first, then your introduction, and finally your supporting points (the body).

The middle section of your essay provides the support for your thesis. This section allows you to highlight your higher-order reasoning skills, and is where you will use the examples from your outline to support your central idea (thesis). An effective essay contains a minimum of three strong examples. Do not jump around between topics in your discussion. Each paragraph must relate to the central thesis presented in your introduction and the sequence of your topics (paragraphs) should build toward a logical conclusion. This is why developing an organizational structure for your essay is one of the keys to writing an effective essay.

Common errors to avoid when composing the body of your essay:

- Avoid making statements based solely on your personal opinion unless you are writing an opinion essay. Even then, you should highlight the evidence that helped you draw your conclusion. In other essay types, you must effectively argue for your thesis; present specific examples that guide your essay to a logical conclusion.
- Don't assume an example is so obvious it doesn't require explanation. Thoroughly explain your examples and always provide enough specifics to enable a reader to appreciate why your example supports your thesis.
- Avoid making global assertions or sweeping generalizations. Remember that your essay should include specifics that can be logically related to one another while exhibiting your critical thinking skills.

HOW ARE ESSAYS GRADED?

Please remember that your response to an essay question demonstrates your ability to (1) understand and interpret directions, (2) recall relevant information, (3) reason, and (4) effectively communicate your thought process in writing. The score that you will be awarded for your response is based on the degree to which your essay reflects these four issues. Just as we recommend that you use an outline to help guide your writing, the individuals that will read (and score) your essay also work from an outline (scoring instruments known as rating scales or grading templates). The criteria used to grade most essays are based on either an analytical or holistic design (Bacha, 2001).

Essay responses are generally graded based on how well your writing sample responds to the task presented. Analytical criteria are used to compare essays from different writers to establish scores; this is norm-referencing (see Chapter 1 for a review). Analytical scoring tends to focus on the details of your essay's structure such as writing style and elements of grammar. In contrast, holistic scoring does not compare essays to each other. Instead, holistic scoring evaluates each essay individually by comparing it against a set of predetermined answer scales; this is criterion-referencing (see Chapter 1 for a discussion of norm- versus criterion-referencing). Holistic scoring focuses more on the organization, completeness, and arrangement of your response than your writing style. Standardized tests generally use holistic scoring instruments to assign a score to your essay.

Holistic grading instruments encourage grading comparability (i.e., minimize the difference in scores between graders). Generally, two readers are assigned to review each essay independently and allot a score based on a comparison of your essay to the predetermined grading rubric. Scores on standardized essays often range in point value from zero to six (in half-point increments) (ETS, 2011; CollegeBoard, 2011; ACT, Inc., 2011).

Your final score will be the average of the scores of the two readers. If the scores of the two readers are markedly different, a third reader is invited to review the essay before a final score is awarded.

AVOID COMMON AND CARELESS ERRORS

A variety of different types of writing errors can lessen the overall effectiveness of your essay, even if it is factually correct or presents a well-reasoned argument. Fortunately, you can learn to write a good essay by simply being aware of common mistakes, learning some basic grammar and style rules, practicing your writing skills beforehand, and, very importantly, *proofreading your essay after you have written it!* Several common writing errors are listed below:

1. Essay response does not address the task posed in the directions.
2. Central idea (thesis) is not clearly stated in the beginning of the essay.
3. Central idea (thesis) is not supported in the body of the essay (e.g., no supporting information is presented, or the information presented is not germane).
4. Essay is rambling and lacking in organization (see previous discussion on the basic structure of an essay and the importance of outlining).

5. Essay contains grammar and punctuation errors (e.g., lack of subject/verb agreement, verb past tense errors, past participle errors, run-on sentences, comma splices, sentence fragments, pronoun errors, misused apostrophes, missing commas, inappropriate verb tense shifts, and misplaced modifiers).
6. Essay contains spelling errors.
7. Essay contains stylistic errors (e.g., use of passive voice, monotonous sentence structure, abrupt transitions, contractions, colloquial expressions, abbreviations, and texting slang).
8. Essay includes exclusionary language (i.e., language that singles out a specific gender, racial, ethnic, or cultural group); avoid this unless it is the topic of your essay (Cengage Learning, 2003).

In summary, when you must respond to an essay question, do the following: (1) read the directions and understand the task, (2) prepare an outline, (3) draft your response by filling in your outline, (4) proofread your essay for errors, and (5) review your essay from the perspective of the reader to make sure you have expressed what you had intended. Always give your essay the polish required to put your best effort forward.

REFERENCES

ACT, Inc. (2011). Scoring guidelines. Retrieved from: http://www. actstudent.org/writing/scores/guidelines.html. Accessed October 11, 2011.

Bacha, N. (2001). Writing evaluation: what can analytic versus holistic essay scoring tell us? *System* 29(3):371–383.

Cengage Learning. (2003). 10 most common grammar errors—and how to avoid them. Retrieved from: http://college.cengage.com/devenglish/ fawcett/evergreen/7e/students/index.html. Accessed October 11, 2011.

CollegeBoard. (2011). Essay scoring guide. Retrieved from: http:// professionals.collegeboard.com/testing/sat-reasoning/scores/essay/ guide. Accessed October 11, 2011.

Davis, B.G., (2009). *Tools for teaching*. San Francisco, CA: Jossey-Bass.

ETS. (2011). How the GRE® tests are scored. Retrieved from: http://www. ets.org/gre/institutions/scores/how/. Accessed October 11, 2011.

Hill, K.L., Hynes G.E., Joyce, M.P., & Green, J.S. (2011). GMAT-AWA score as a predictor of success in a managerial communication course. *Business Communication Quarterly* 74(2):103–118.

Moss, A. & Holder, C. (1988). *Improving student learning.* Dubuque, IA: Kendall/Hunt.

Reiner, C.M., Bothell, T.W., Sudweeks, R.R., & Wood, B. (2002). *Preparing effective essay questions.* Stillwater, OK: New Forums Press.

References

ACT, Inc. (2011). Scoring guidelines. Retrieved from: http://www.actstudent. org/writing/scores/guidelines.html. Accessed October 11, 2011.

Ambose, S.A., Bridges, M.W., Lovett, M.C., DiPietro, M., & Norman, M.K. (2010). *How learning works: 7 Research-based principles for smart teachers.* San Francisco, CA: Jossey-Bass.

Association of American Publishers. (2011). Standardized assessment: A primer. Washington DC. Retrieved from: http://aapschool.org/pdf/ Testing%20Primer%20Revised.pdf. Accessed October 11, 2011.

Bacha, N. (2001). Writing evaluation: what can analytic versus holistic essay scoring tell us? *System* 29(3):371–383.

Bangert-Drowns, R.L., Kulik, J.A., & Kulik, C.L. (1983). Effects of coaching programs on achievement test performance. *Review of Educational Research* 53:571–585.

Barlow, D. (2002). *Anxiety and its disorders* (2nd ed.). New York: Guilford Press.

Benjamin, L.T., Cavell, T.A., & Shallenberger, W.R. (2984). Staying with initial answers on objective tests—Is it a myth? *Teaching of Psychology* 11:133–141.

Benjamin, M., McKeachie, W.J., Lin, Y., & Holinger, D.P. (1981). Test anxiety: Deficits in information processing. *Journal of Educational Psychology* 73(6):816–824.

Benson, H. (1985). *Beyond the relaxation response.* New York: Berkley Books.

Bice, G. & Sefcik, D. (2010). CME: What works for me. *Clinician Reviews* 20(1):3.

Birenbaum, M. & Nasser, F. (1994). On the relationship between test anxiety and test performance. *Measurement and Evaluation in Counseling and Development* 27(1):293–301.

Board, C. & Whitney, D.R. (1972). The effect of selected poor item-writing practices on test difficulty, reliability and validity. *Research Report 55,* University Evaluation and Examination Service, University of Iowa.

Boekaerts, M. (1997). Self-regulated learning: A new concept embraced by researchers, policy makers, educators, teachers, and students. *Learning and Instruction* 7(2):161–186.

Brewer, T. (2002). Test taking anxiety among nursing students and general college students. *Journal of Psychosocial Nursing* 40(11):23–29.

Brockkamp, H. & Van Hout-Wolters, B.H.A.M. (2007). Students' adaption of study strategies when preparing for classroom tests. *Educational Psychological Reviews* 19:401–428.

Burns, D.J. (2008). Will I do as well on the first exam as I expect? An examination of students' expectations. *Journal of the Scholarship of Teaching and Learning*. 8(3):1–19.

Cengage Learning. (2003). 10 most common grammar errors—and how to avoid them. Retrieved from: http://college.cengage.com/devenglish/ fawcett/evergreen/7e/students/index.html. Accessed October 11, 2011.

Chapell, M., Blanding, Z., Silverstein M., & Gubi, A. (2005). Test anxiety and academic performance in undergraduate and graduate students. *Journal of Educational Psychology* 97(2):268–274.

Chaplin, S. (2007). A model of student success: Coaching students to develop critical thinking skills in introductory biology courses. *International Journal for the Scholarship of Teaching and Learning* 1(2): 1–7.

Coderre, S., Woloschuk, W., & McLaughlin, K. (2009). Twelve tips for blueprinting. *Medical Teacher* 31:322–324.

Coffield, F.J., Moseley, D.V., Hall E., & Ecclestone, K. (2004). *Learning styles and pedagogy in post-16 learning: A systematic and critical review.* London: Learning and Skills Research Centre.

CollegeBoard. (2011). Essay scoring guide. Retrieved from: http:// professionals.collegeboard.com/testing/sat-reasoning/scores/essay/ guide. Accessed October 11, 2011.

Colvin, G. (2010). *Talent is overrated.* New York: Penguin Group.

Crooks, T.J. (1988). The impact of classroom evaluation practices on students. *Review of Educational Research* 58(4):438–481.

Croskerry, P. (2003). The importance of cognitive errors in diagnosis and strategies to minimize them. *Academic Medicine* 78:775–780.

Davis, B.G. (2009). *Tools for teaching.* San Francisco, CA: Jossey-Bass.

Davis, M., Eshelman, E.R., & McKay, M. (2000). *The relaxation and stress reduction workbook.* Oakland CA: New Harbinger Publications.

Diamond, J.J. & Evans, W.J. (1972). An investigation of the cognitive correlates of test-wiseness. *Journal of Educational Measurement* 9: 145–150.

Dickinson, D.J. & O'Connell, D.Q. (1990). Using test-taking strategies to maximize multiple-choice test scores. *Journal of Educational Research* 83(4):227–230.

Dolly, J.P. & Williams, K.S. (1986). Using test-taking strategies to maximize multiple-choice test scores. *Educational and Psychological Measurement* 46:619–265.

Duckworth, A.L. & Seligman, M.E.P. (2005). Self-discipline outdoes IQ in predicting academic performance of adolescents. *Psychological Science* 16(12):939–944.

Ellis, Y., Daniels, B., & Jauregui, A. (2010). The effect of multitasking on the grade performance of business students. *Research in Higher Education Journal* 8. Retrieved from: http://www.aabri.com/manuscripts/10498.pdf. Accessed October 11, 2011.

Ergene, T. (2003). Effective interventions on test anxiety reduction: A meta analysis. *School Psychology International* 24(3):313–320.

Ericsson, K.A., Prietula, M.J., & Cokely, E.T. (2007). The making of an expert. *Harvard Business Review* 2007 (July-August):115–121.

ETS. (2011). How the GRE® tests are scored. Retrieved from: http://www.ets.org/gre/institutions/scores/how/. Accessed October 11, 2011.

Eva, K.W., Norman, G.R., & Neville, A.J., Wood, T.J., & Brooks, L.R. (2002). Expert-novice differences in memory: A reformulation. *Teaching and Learning in Medicine* 14(4):257–263.

Evans, W. (1984). Test wiseness: An examination of cue-using strategies. *Journal of Experimental Education* 52(3):141–144.

Fanning, P. (1994). *Visualization for change.* Oakland CA: New Harbinger Publications.

Gall, M. (1984). Synthesis of research on teachers' questioning. *Educational Leadership* 42(3):40–47.

Gerhardt, M.W. & Luzadais, R.A. (2009). The importance of perceived task difficulty in goal orientation—Assigned goal alignment. *Journal of Leadership and Organizational Studies* 16(2):167–174.

Gurung, R.A.R. (2005). How do students really study (and does it matter)? *Teaching of Psychology* 32(4):238–240.

Gurung, R.A.R., Weidert, J., & Jeske, A. (2010). Focusing on how students study. *Journal of the Scholarship of Teaching and Learning* 10(1):28–35.

Haladyna, T.M. (2004). *Developing and validating multiple-choice test items.* Mahwah, NJ: Erlbaum.

Hayes, J. (1989). *The complete problem solver.* Hillsdale, NJ: Erlbaum.

Helmstetter, S. (1987). *The self-talk solution.* New York: Pocket Books.

Helmstetter, S. (1990). *The self-talk solution.* New York: Pocket Books.

Hill K.L., Hynes G.E., Joyce, M.P., & Green J.S. (2011). GMAT-AWA score as a predictor of success in a managerial communication course. *Business Communication Quarterly* 74(2):103–118.

Hong, E. & Karstensson, L. (2002). Antecedents of state test anxiety. *Contemporary Educational Psychology* 27:348–367.

Hopko, D., Hunt, M., & Armento, M. (2005). Attentional task aptitude and performance anxiety. *International Journal of Stress Management* 12(4):389–408.

Jandaghi, G. & Shaterian, F. (2008). Validity, reliability and difficulty indices for instructor-built exam questions. *Journal of Applied Quantitative Methods* 3(2):151–155.

Johns, J.L. & McNamara, L.P. (1980). The SQ3R study technique: A forgotten research target. *Journal of Reading* 23(8):705–708.

Johnson, S. (2000). *Taking the anxiety out of taking tests: A step by step guide.* New York: Barnes and Noble Books.

Karpicke, J.D., Butler, A.C., & Roediger, H.L. (2009). Metacognitive strategies in student learning: Do students practice retrieval when they study on their own? *Memory* 17, 471–479.

Kempainen, R.P., Migeon, M.B., & Wolf, F.M. (2003). Understanding our mistakes: A primer on errors in clinical reasoning. *Medical Teacher* 25(2):177–181.

King, A. (1992). Comparison of self-questioning, summarizing, and notetaking-review as strategies for learning from lectures. *American Educational Research Journal* 29(2):303–323.

Kitsantas, A. (2002). Test preparation and performance: A self-regulatory analysis. *Journal of Experimental Education* 70(2):101–113.

Krause, L.B. (2003). *How we learn and why we don't* (4th Ed.). Mason, OH: Thomson Custom Publishing.

Kruger, J. & Dunning, D. (1999). Unskilled and unaware of it: How difficulties in recognizing one's own incompetence lead to inflated self-assessments. *Journal of Personality and Social Psychology* 77(6):1121–1134.

Kruger, J., Wirtz, D., & Miller, D.T. (2005). Counterfactual thinking and the first instinct fallacy. *Journal of Personality and Social Psychology* 88(5):725–735.

Kuncel, N.R. & Hezlett, S.A. (2007). Standardized tests predict graduate students' success. *Science* 315:1080–1081.

Laatsch, L. (2009). Evaluation and treatment of students with difficulties passing the step examinations. *Academic Medicine* 84(5):677–683.

Lai, E.R. & Waltman, K. (2008). Test preparation: Examining teacher perceptions and practices. *Educational Measurement: Issues and Practice* 27(2):28–45.

Larsen, J. (2006). A Resource for USMLE step 1 preparation. Retrieved from: http://www.ttuhsc.edu/som/studentaffairs/documents/Step_1_ Prep_Book.pdf. Accessed October 11, 2011.

Ley, K. & Young, D.B. (2001). Instructional principles for self-regulation. *Educational Technology Research and Development* 49(2):93–101.

Mahamed, A., Gregory, P.A.M., & Austin, A. (2006). "Testwiseness" among international pharmacy graduates and Canadian senior pharmacy students. *American Journal of Pharmaceutical Education* 70(6):131.

Mason, J. (1985). *Guide to stress reduction.* Berkeley, CA: Celestial Arts.

Mayer, R.E. (2010). Applying the science of learning to medical education. *Medical Education* 44:543–549.

McIntyre, S.H. & Munson, J.M. (2008). Exploring cramming: Student behaviors, beliefs, and learning retention in the principles of marketing course. *Journal of Marketing Education* 30(3):226–243.

McKay, M., Davis, M., & Fanning, P. (1998). *Thoughts and feelings The art of cognitive stress reduction.* Oakland CA: New Harbinger Publications.

Medina, J. (2008). *Brain rules.* Seattle, WA: Pear Press.

Michael, J. (2006). Where's the evidence that active learning works? *Advances in Physiology Education* 30:159–167.

Milman, J., Bishop, C.H., & Ebel, R. (1965). An analysis of test-wiseness. *Educational and Psychological Measurement* 25(3):707–726.

Millman, J. (1969). *How to take tests.* New York: McGraw-Hill.

Morse, D.T. (1998). The relative difficulty of selected test-wiseness skills among college students. *Educational and Psychological Measurement* 58(3):399–408.

Moss, A. & Holder, C. (1988). *Improving student learning.* Dubuque, IA: Kendall/Hunt.

Mueller, J. (1980). Test anxiety and the encoding and retrieval of information. In I. Sarason, *Test anxiety: Theory, research and applications.* Hillside: Erlbaum.

Myers, I.B., McCaulley, M.H., Quenk, N.L., & Hammer, A.L. (1998). *MBTI Manual: A guide to the development and use of the Myers-Briggs Type Indicator* (3rd ed.). Palo Alto, CA: Consulting Psychologists Press.

Pekrun, R., Goetz, T., Titz, W., & Perry, R.P. (2002). Academic emotions in students' self-regulated learning and achievement: A program of quantitative and qualitative research. *Educational Psychologist* 37:91–106.

Pelley, J.W. & Dalley, B.K. (2008). *Success types for medical students: A program for improving academic performance.* Lubbock, TX: Texas Tech University Division of Extended Studies.

Poorman, S. & Webb, C. (2000). Preparing to retake the NCLEX-RN: The experience of graduates who fail. *Nurse Educator* 25(4):175–180.

Rackman, N. (1979). The coaching controversy. *Training and Development Journal* 33(11):12–16.

Regehr, G. & Eva, K. (2006). Self-assessment, self-direction and the self-regulating professional. *Clinical Orthopaedics and Related Research* 449:34–38.

Reiner, C.M., Bothell, T.W., Sudweeks, R.R., & Wood, B. (2002). *Preparing Effective Essay Questions*. Stillwater, OK: New Forums Press.

Robinson, F. (1970). *Effective study*. New York: Harper & Row.

Rubenstein, J.S., Meyer, D.E., & Evans, J.E. (2001). Executive control of cognitive processes in task switching. *Journal of Experimental Psychology* 27(4):763–797.

Samson, G.E. (1985). Effects of training in test-taking skills on achievement test performance: A quantitative synthesis. *Journal of Educational Research* 78(5):261–266.

Sarnacki, R.E. (1979). An examination of test-wiseness in the cognitive test domain. *Review of Educational Research* 49(2):252–279.

Schultz, P. & Davis, H. (2000). Emotions and self-regulation during test taking. *Educational Psychologist* 35:243–256.

Scruggs, T.E. & Mastropieri, M.A. (1992). *Teaching test-taking skills*. Cambridge, MA: Brookline Books.

Sefcik, D.J. & Obi, P. (2005). *The value of a commercial test-preparation course on COMLEX. Level 1 performance*. Poster presented at the 3rd annual meeting of the American Association of Colleges of Osteopathic Medicine, Bethesda, MD.

Sefcik, D.J. & Prerost, F.J. (2001). *The impact of review course participation on preparation for the PANC*. Paper presented at the Annual Education Forum of the Association of Physician Assistant Programs, Albuquerque, NM.

Sefcik, D.J., Prerost, F.J., & Arbet, S.E. (2009). Personality types and performance on aptitude and achievement tests: Implications for osteopathic educators. *Journal of the American Osteopathic Association* 2009;109(6):296–301.

Shirom, A., Toker, S., Alkaly, Y., Jacobson, O., & Balicer, R. (2011). Work-based predictors of mortality: A 20-year follow-up of healthy employees. *Health Psychology* 30(3):268–275.

Shrock, S. & Coscarelli, W. (2000). *Criterion-referenced test development.* Silver Springs, MD: International Society for Performance Improvement.

Sideridis, G.D. (2005). Goal orientation, academic achievement, and depression: Evidence in favor of a revised goal theory framework. *Journal of Educational Psychology* 97(3):366–375.

Simpson, M.L. & Nist, S.L. (2000). An update on strategic learning: It's more than textbook reading strategies. *Journal of Adolescent & Adult Literacy* 43(6):528–541.

Slakter, M.J., Koehler, R.A., & Hampton, S.H. (1970). Learning test-wiseness by programmed texts. *Journal of Educational Measurement* 7(4):247–254.

Smith, J.K. (1982). Converging on correct answers: A peculiarity of multiple choice items. *Journal of Educational Measurement* 3:211–220.

Sousa, D.A. (2006). *How the brain learns* (3rd ed.). Thousand Oaks, CA: Corwin Press.

Speizer, I. (2005). Value-minded. *Workforce Management* 84:55–58.

Spielberger, C. & Vagg, P. (1995). *Test anxiety: Theory, assessment and treatment.* Bristol PA: Taylor and Francis.

Spielberger, D. (1985). Anxiety, cognition, and affect: A state-trait perspective. In A. Tuma & J. Maser, Eds., *Anxiety, and the anxiety disorders.* Hillside, NJ: Erlbaum.

Thomas, E.L. & Robinson, H.A. (1982). *Improving reading in every classroom: A source book for teachers.* Boston: Allyn & Bacon.

Tigner, R.B. (1999). Putting memory research to good use: Hints from cognitive psychology. *College Teaching* 47(4):149–151.

Townsend, D.J. & Bever, T.G. (2001). *Sentence comprehension the integration of habits and rules.* Cambridge, MA: MIT Press.

Veenman, M., Keseboom, L., & Imthorn, C. (2000). Test anxiety and metacognitive skillfulness: Availability versus production deficiencies. *Anxiety, Stress and Coping* 13(4):391–413.

Weber, C. & Bizer, G. (2005). The effects of immediate forewarning of test difficulty on test performance. *Journal of General Psychology* 133(3):277–285.

West, D.C., Pomeroy, J.R., Park, J.K., Gerstenberger, E.A., & Sandoval, J. (2000). Critical thinking in graduate medical education. A role for concept mapping? *JAMA* 284(9):1105–1110.

Winne, P.H. & Nesbit, J.C. (2010). The psychology of academic achievement. *Annual Review of Psychology* 61:653–678.

Wood, W. & Neal, D.T. (2007). A new look at habits and the habit-goal interface. *Psychological Review* 114(4): 843–863.

Zheng, A.Y., Lawhorn, J.K., Lumley, T., & Freeman, S. (2008). Application of Bloom's taxonomy debunks the "MCAT myth." *Science* 319:414–415.

Zimmerman, B.J. & Pons, M.M. (1986). Development of a structured interview for assessing student use of self-regulated learning strategies. *American Educational Research Journal* 23(4):614–628.

Index

"should" statements, 189
similar alternatives, in MCQs, 162
six-step approach to reading,
    117–118
skills
    in test blueprint, 22
    test-taking. *See* test-taking skills
skills deficit issue, 173–174, 184–186
sleep, 77, 150, 181–182
SMART goals, 63
S-N (Sensing-Intuition) dichotomy,
    50–51
social support network, 78–79
spaced studying, 72
Speizer, I., xxi
spelling errors, 211
SQ4R reading technique, 116–118
ST (sensing-thinking) mental function
    types, 50–51, 136–137
stamina maintenance, 150–151
standardized tests
    activity, 13–14
    features of, 5–6
    teacher-generated tests vs., 7–9
    websites for, 199–201
stem component, of test questions,
    122–123, 158
stimulus-response, 93
strategy, defined, 105
stresses, of timed environment,
    143–144
study aids
    complex, 99–100
    defined, 48, 52
    illusion of competence with, 97–98
    mnemonics, 96–97
    Q&A resources, 54–55
    for qualitative learning, 98–99
    review courses, 53–54
    selection of, xix
    simple, 99
    traditional/review books, 53
study behaviors
    categories of, 55–57
    defined, 48

evaluation exercise, xxiii–xxv
    memory and, 96
    selection of, xix
study for recall, 93–95
study plans
    drafting exercise, xxi–xxiii
    finalizing exercise, 196–198
study resources
    activity, 58
    defined, 48
    flexibility and, 51–52
    illusion of competence and, 97–98
    overview, 47
    personality/preferences and, 48–51
    selecting, 52–57
study schedules
    development of master, 70–72
    format of, 69–70
    importance of, 67–69
    to-do lists vs., 72–73
study systems, for reducing anxiety,
    185–186
stylistic errors, 211
subconscious behaviors, 30
success, 35, 36–38
summarizing, as study behavior, 56
superficial learning strategies. *See* lower-
    level learning
support, 78–79
survey stage, of reading skills, 116–117
switch tasking, 89
synthesis essays, 205

T

table of specifications. *See* test blue-
    prints
tables, as study aids, 100
tactics, of low-performing students,
    105
taking responsibility, 36–38
Taking the Anxiety Out of Taking Tests
    (Johnson), 188
tardiness, time management and, 60
teacher-generated tests, 7–9
TEAMS approach, xix, 27–28